THE SIRTFOOD DIET FOR BEGINNE~

**7-Day Meal Plan to Activate Your Skinny Gene and Burn Fat.
28 Days Program to Stay Fit and Healthy With
Original Sirt Recipes**

Adele Goggins

Table of Contents

INTRODUCTION

The Sirtfood diet targets eating foods full of sirtuin proteins sirt1 - sirt7. Sirtuins are proven to contribute to glucose and fat metabolic rate regulation in reaction to fluctuations in energy. These proteins additionally impact calorie restriction on developments in aging. The diet is consequently believed to influence your human body's ability to burn off fat and enhances the metabolic process.

What the dietary plan entails

The diet carries a weekly program. Within the first three days, calories are restricted to 1000 calories per day. Those calories include three Sirtfood green juices, along with a typical meal that's composed of Sirtfood.

After which, calories are raised to 1,500 per day. Throughout this time, dieters drink just two juices and also consume two meals every day.

What foods you can eat

The diet necessitates its followers to consume foods that are full of sirtuins.

Such foods include:

- Chocolate

- Red wine

- Kale

- Blueberries

- Citrus fruits

- Prawns

- Salmons

The diet additionally requires visitors to drink green juices extracted from foods full of sirtuins, such as ginseng, citrus and strawberry.

Moreover, research indicates that transgenic mice with significantly high rates of sirt6 live somewhat longer than mice in the wild, thus purporting the belief that sirt6 could affect the aging of several human cells. Sirt2 additionally was demonstrated to impede metazoan aging.

Additionally, these results sound impressive along with the dietary plan's glowing reviews, but this does not reflect a persuasive scientific proof about the effects of the diet providing similar results in real men and women.

Furthermore, it is good to assume that lab research conducted on yeast, mice and human stem cells were tainted since there are many variables to consider.

The science of fat reduction

Indeed, the diet will probably seem to work with a lot of people. However, scientific evidence of any diet's success is a rather different issue. The perfect study in relation to the efficacy of a daily diet for fat loss or another outcome – for example, reduce the symptoms of aging might necessitate a sufficiently large sample – representative of the populace – and also an arbitrary allocation to your control or treatment group.

Outcomes would subsequently be tracked over a reasonable time period with strict control of confounding variables, such as with other behaviors that will positively or negatively impact the results – for example, smoking or physical exercise.

Research of this aspect is not possible and we all have to consequently be wary with the interpretation of fundamental science - all things considered, human cells within a tissue culture dish likely respond differently to the tissues of a living person.

Further doubt arises about the effectiveness of this particular diet once we consider a number of particular claims:

Losses of pounds in one week are both unrealistic and, therefore, are rather unlikely to reveal changes to human body fat loss. In the initial three days of the diet, dieters eat up around 1000 calories - approximately 40 to 50 percent of exactly what a lot of men and women require. This can create an instant loss in glycogen a stored form of carbohydrate from visceral fat and the liver.

- However, for each and every gram of glycogen, we additionally store approximately 2.7 g of water. Thus, for many of the glycogen, we also lose excess fat and thus, weight.

- In addition, diets that are too restrictive have become hard to consistently follow and lead to gains in appetite-stimulating hormones, such as ghrelin.

- Weight water and glycogen will consequently return if the impulse to eat increases after the restrictive phase.

- Additionally, it is usually not feasible to implement placebo-controlled trials that have any level of ecological validity, and also medical effects we tend to be interested to perform over many decades, which makes research seem difficult.

- Moreover, studies in huge populations rely on amazingly simplistic and basic data collection techniques like memory and also self-reporting that produce infamously unreliable data. Against this background, nutrition research is a challenging task.

Can anything be done to fix this?

Regrettably, this may not be possible. Sensationalized headlines and frequently blatant representation of scientific data ends in the apparently endless controversies by exactly what and how much. We can eat, further afield our obsession with a "quick fix" or miracle cure that is an endemic social issue.

The Sirtfood diet ought to be consigned into the trend heap - from the scientific standpoint. To get the reasons summarized, the Sirtfood dietary plan needs to be consigned into the trend heap - from the scientific perspective.

According to the evidence we've to indicate otherwise. They are at best spurious and in worst ineffective and damaging to the true goal of a community health plan. The diet is not likely to provide any advantage to people facing an epidemic of diabetes, even culminating in the gloom of obesity.

As stated quite plainly by many others, special diet plans usually don't work and dieting generally isn't really a general health solution for societies in which over fifty percent of adults are overweight.

Currently, the very best strategy is long-term behavior shift together with environmental and political sway, geared toward improved physical activity along with some sort of control over what we eat. It is perhaps not a fast fix; however, it is going to get the job done.

WHAT IS SIRTFOOD DIET?

The Sirt diet consists of two phases that last a total of three weeks. If you hope to lose more weight, then you can repeat these two phases in turn until you reach your goal weight. It's important that you do this, rather than lengthening the first phase, as the phases must be combined as intended for healthy weight loss. This is because the first phase, which lasts one week, reduces your kilocalorie intake, and the second phase is needed to balance this reduction. If you lengthen the first phase, you will not be offering your body the full nutrition it needs in the second phase. So, always remember, the first phase should never last longer than a week, and it should always be followed with the second phase. Now, let's examine these two phases.

During both phases of the diet, you will be drinking the signature Sirt green juice. The reason that this juice is important is that it offers you a number of sirtfoods in a concentrated form, activating your body's weight loss potential and boosting your health. This juice is an integral part of the diet, and can't be skipped over. Thankfully, with just a few ingredients, you can easily make this juice in only a few minutes a day. I recommend making this juice first thing in the morning so that you always start your day by revving up your metabolism and boosting fat loss. While you will need multiple servings of green juice throughout the day, you can make it all in the morning and store what you will drink later in the day in the fridge, so that you only have to prepare it once a day. While it may be tempting to make all of your green juice at the beginning of the week, sadly, this is not an option. The reason for this is because science has found that after you make juice, every day that it is stored, it will lose an increasing number of nutrients. Due to this, you should never make your green juice more than one day in advance.

How does the Sirtfood diet work?

Phase One:

The first phase of the Sirt diet lasts seven days. During this time, your kilocalories will be greatly reduced, and you will drink an increased amount of green juice a day to really push you to lose weight. This reduced kilocalorie intake is precisely controlled so that you stay healthy and still consume the nutrients your body requires. This phase is when you will lose the most weight, especially the first time you complete this phase as you will not only be losing fat, but also water weight.

In the first three days of this phase, you will be consuming one-thousand kilocalories per day. Days four through seven will include an increase to fifteen-hundred kilocalories a day. But, it is not all about restricting kilocalories, but also increasing nutrition and sirtfoods. Therefore, you will also be drinking three servings of green juice a day and, on average, eating two to three meals depending on how many kilocalories they contain.

While red wine is a classic Sirtfood, it is only consumed after phase one. This is because the alcohol may hinder your weight loss if you drink it during the first phase, and due to your reduced kilocalorie intake, you could experience more intense side effects from drinking.

Phase Two:

After the rapid weight loss in phase one, the second phase is designed to keep up your progress with weight maintenance. In this phase, your caloric intake is not reduced. You can freely consume; however, many kilocalories are recommended according to your BMI or body-mass index and activity level. If you don't know your personal caloric recommendation, then you can easily find a BMI calculator online or ask your doctor.

You will continue to drink one serving of green juice daily, along with balanced healthy meals full of sirtfoods. The recipes in this guidelines work for both phases of the diet, and you can simply eat; however, much is needed for your kilocalorie intake on a given day. But, you can also customize your favorite family recipes by including more sirtfoods in them. For instance, if your family loves pizza, then why not try adding some buckwheat to the crust and topping it with some onion, kale, and soy-based bacon replacement? By making pizza in this way, you can get four different types of sirtfoods. Of course, you shouldn't only consume sirtfoods. A healthy and balanced diet requires foods from all over the produce department, so make sure you eat a variety of fresh fruits and vegetables.

While the first phase lasts one week, the second phase lasts two weeks, or you can continue this phase indefinitely. Remember, if you want to increase your weight loss from the first phase, don't lengthen that phase. Instead, continue following both weeks of phase two, and then you can repeat phases one and two in turn. This will ensure you lose weight in a healthy and maintainable way.

Is this diet really healthy?

Sirtfoods are mostly all healthy options as well as could also lead to some health advantages as a result of their antioxidant or anti-inflammatory homes. Yet consuming merely a handful of specifically healthy foods can not satisfy every one of your body s nutritional demands. The Sirtfood Diet is unnecessarily limiting as well as uses no clear, special wellness benefits over any other sort of diet regimen. Furthermore, consuming simply 1,000 calories is normally not advised without the guidance of a doctor. Even consuming 1,500 calories daily is extremely restrictive for numerous individuals.

The diet likewise needs draining to 3 green juices every day. Although juices can be an exceptional source of minerals and vitamins, they are likewise a source of sugar and also consist of virtually none of the healthy fiber that whole veggies and also fruits do.

Who is This Diet Suitable for?

1. You know that you have overindulged during the holidays, but as you weigh yourself, you literally would want to shave all the extra pounds because you did not expect to have gained that much weight!

2. There is an upcoming wedding event, and you need to lose those extra pounds in

order to fit your into your gown/suit. There is no way that you are going to lose that much weight in 2 months!

3. You know that you are overweight and just plain unhealthy. You have already tried a number of diets, but to no avail. Either you feel that those diets are too restrictive, there is an adverse health effect, and the diet is too expensive to maintain. Speaking of maintenance, you are having a hard time to keep off the little weight that you have managed to loose!

4. You are getting older and you start to notice that aside from having a hard time dealing with hangovers and late night parties, losing and maintaining weight is not that easy as it used to be. You are not a big fan of eliminating numerous food groups and doing rigorous exercise.

You have probably heard these scenarios to many times before and you have probably experienced one or two, or you are in one of these scenarios right now. Being overweight or obese is actually one of the most common health problems around the world. According to the World Health Organization, being overweight is when your BMI is equal to or greater than 25, while being obese is when your BMI is equal to or greater than 30.

In the 2014 data from WHO, worldwide obesity has more than doubled since 1980, and more than 1.9 billion adults are overweight; and it would safe to conclude that after two years that that number has already increased significantly.

Health experts agree that this is a very alarming rate, but the good news is, obesity or having excess weight is preventable and reversible.

As you will notice, most of these scenarios are focused on the aesthetics looking good and feeling more confident about your body, but what I would like to stress is the ill-effects of every extra bulge or pound that we carry. The possible health illnesses associated with being overweight is the primary reason why you need to try the revolutionary Sirtfood diet.

Given everything that you have learned about the Sirtfood Diet, the most important question—at least for many people—is whether or not it is worth your time and effort.

If you were to listen to its celebrity endorsers, such as food writer and TV chef Lorraine Pascale, then you hear a lot about how the diet has helped them lose weight, enhance their muscles, and feel better about themselves.

However, some skeptics of this diet argue that these may have been the combined effects of other weight loss measures and fitness regimes that these celebrities follow. After all, many of them have easy access to personal trainers and dieticians.

So, for an average woman who has relatively limited means, would the Sirtfood Diet still work just as well?

From a scientific point of view, multiple studies conducted using animal subjects support the claim about the weight loss capabilities of certain sirtfoods, especially blueberries and grapes.

Though the findings of this trial have proven to be quite promising, other experts have noted certain limitations of the study that could have been improved upon if subsequent follow-up trials had been conducted. Some of the most prominent limitations identified include the following:

- Lack of control group to as serve as baseline and reference point;

- Having 40 participants only, which is relatively small sample size; and

- Probable bias among the participants, since they have been identified as health-conscious individuals.

These limitations, while not conclusive, somehow weaken foundations of the Sirtfood Diet. Some health experts even argue that much like other types of diets, Sirtfood Diet could help its followers lose weight by imposing caloric limits for a certain period.

While restrictive eating can be helpful and effective to a certain extent, several studies have highlighted the negative impacts that this practice causes. If you have already tried doing diets that are centered around regular fasting, then you would have experienced mood swings, sudden binges to compensate for the lack of food, loss of muscle mass and strength, and even depression.

Granted that you will not be required to undergo special exercise routines or to cut back on different types of food, you would still have to be mindful of what you eat and drink while you are on the Sirtfood diet. Nonetheless, this level of leniency that this diet offers to attract a lot of people who do not want to give up a lot of things for the sake of looking and feeling better.

So, what's the verdict on the Sirtfood Diet?

If you are willing to live through its drawbacks to reap its benefits and enjoy its advantages over other weight loss plans, then, go ahead with your plans to follow this diet. This book has shed light on what to expect and what you should do to successfully finish both of its phases.

Furthermore, the majority of the top sirtfoods are fruits, vegetables, and plant-based foods. When combined with the right amount of proteins and carbohydrates in your daily meals, then you cannot go wrong by eating more of them than you usually do. Just remember to keep your red wine, caffeine, and dark chocolate in moderation though, to avoid causing unintentional harm to your body.

Finally, as a rule of thumb, you should not put your 100% trust on a diet that has promises that sound a bit too good to be true. Set realistic expectations based on your current situation in life. Not everyone can live like Adele and the other celebrity endorsers of the Sirtfood Diet.

WHAT IS THE SKINNY GENE?

Sirtuins are also often called the Skinny Gene because of the role they can play in reducing human weight. But how these genes can make that magic happen is an important question. Biological sciences are no magic, it's all about understanding your body better and then meeting the body's needs to help boost its natural healthy activities. Similarly, when we boost the formation and stimulation of sirtuins in the cell, it automatically aids metabolism, prevents aging, and puts the body on a fast track.

Not every person is obese due to lack of exercise or the food they eat some people have a naturally low metabolic rate and it makes it almost impossible for them to get out of the trap of obesity. By stimulating the sirtuins, we can put the body on track and make burning calories faster and use them effectively.

Fasting-based diets have become very popular over the past few years. In fact, studies show that by fasting - that is, with moderate daily calorie restriction or by practicing a more radical, but less frequent intermittent fast - you can expect to lose about six pounds in six months and substantially reduce the risk of contracting certain diseases.

The accumulation of fat stops and the body blocks normal growth processes and enters "survival" mode. Fats are burned faster and the genes that repair and rejuvenate cells are activated. As a result, we lose weight and increase our resistance to disease.

The mysteries of thinness

Many studies have looked at the genetic specificities of overweight or obese people, Sadaf Farooqi, professor at the University of Cambridge, has chosen to focus on those of thin people. For this research, Sadaf Farroqi and his team worked with 1,622 thin volunteers, and used data from 1,985 severely obese people and 10,433 people of normal weight. Their DNA was collected and they answered a questionnaire on their state of health and their lifestyle.

Slimming is linked to genetics

The DNA study confirmed the results of studies: certain genes have a role in the risk of obesity and have allowed new discoveries to be made, in particular that other genes seem to be involved in slimming. The researchers gathered the data collected to develop a genetic risk index. "As we imagined, we found that obese people have a higher genetic risk index than people with normal weight," said one of the study authors. Conversely, thin people have a lower genetic risk index. 74% of the slim people in the study had slim and healthy people in their genealogy.

Target these genes to avoid obesity

"It's easy to make hasty judgments and criticize people for their weight, but science shows that things are much more complex, says Sadaf Farooqi. He now wants to push his research to identify precisely which gene influences thinness, this could help put the weight of specific treatment strategies for overweight people.

All this, however, has a price. Lower energy intake leads to hunger, irritability, exhaustion and loss of muscle mass. And the problem is precisely this with fasting-based diets: when they are followed correctly, they work, but they make us feel so bad that we cannot respect them. The question, then, is the following: is it possible to obtain the same results without having to impose that drastic drop in calories and, therefore, without suffering the negative consequences?

Although Sirt foods are not a mainstay of nutrition in England today, the situation was quite different in the past. They were a basic element, and if many have become rare and others have even disappeared, we will soon see that it is possible to reverse the course.

For the first time, researchers have just highlighted a genetic cause of pathological thinness, associated with a risk of high mortality.

These studies, which point to the role of excess genes in underweight people who have difficulty eating, are published on Wednesday by the British scientific journal Nature.

The study, which involved 100,000 people, was led by Philippe Froguel Imperial College / London and Institute Pasteur de Lille / France and the Swiss team of Jacques Beckmann University of Lausanne.

A fragment of chromosome 16 is known to be sometimes subject to fluctuations in the number of copies of its genes. The vast majority of people have two copies of each gene in this part of the chromosome, one transmitted by the mother, the other by the father. But about one in 2,500 people has only one copy an under-dosage and one in 2,000 has three copies overdose of genes.

The Franco-Anglo-Swiss team had discovered in 2010 that the presence of a whole a single copy in this fragment of chromosome 16 could explain 1% of severe obesity.

It now demonstrates that people with an excess of genetic material and therefore having three copies of this part of chromosome 16 have significant, even extreme thinness. They are up to 20 times more likely to be underweight than the general population.

Foods that activate sirtuins

Turmeric and Kale are Sirtfoods and as indicated by analysts, these uncommon nourishments work by enacting explicit proteins in the body called sirtuins. Sirtuins are accepted to shield cells in the body from kicking the bucket when they are under pressure and are thought to manage irritation, digestion and the maturing procedure. Analysts likewise accept sirtuins impact the body's capacity to consume fat and lift digestion.

Top 10 Sirtfoods and others

When on a Sirtfood diet, you have to make sure that most of the following ingredients are in your meal plan:

1. Arugula rocket
2. Bird's eye chili
3. Blueberries
4. Buckwheat
5. Capers
6. Celery
7. Coffee
8. Dark chocolate 85% cocoa or cocoa
9. Extra-virgin olive oil
10. Kale

Perhaps, other people might be thinking, "What kind of diet is this? Red wine and dark chocolate? It simply doesn't make any sense." As it turns out, it does. Scientifically speaking, the ingredients above are the richest in sirtuins, so it is highly recommended to consume them. However, moderate consumption is recommended, as you don't need to get drunk on red wine to get the sirtuins you need.

Moreover, you don't have to consume just these ingredients, as there aren't too many recipes of food made only from them. After all, this is what the sirtuin diet is about combining calorie restriction with sirtfoods, not just to eat food rich in this class of proteins.

Let's take them one by one to learn a bit more about them.

HOW TO FOLLOW THE SIRTDIET

Starting the Sirtfood diet is very easy. It just takes a bit of preparation. If you do not know what Kale is, or where you would find Green Tea, then you may have a learning curve, albeit very small. There is little in the way of starting the Sirtfood diet.

Since you will be preparing and cooking healthy foods, you may want to do a few things the week you start:

1. Clear your cabinets and refrigerator of foods that are obviously unhealthy and that might tempt you. You also will have a very low calorie intake at the start, and you do not want to be tempted into a quick fix that may set you back. Even though you will have new recipes, you may feel that your old comfort foods are easier at the moment.

2. Go shopping for all of the ingredients that you will need for the week. If you buy what you will need it is more cost effective. Also, once you see the recipes, you will notice that there are many ingredients that overlap. You will get to know your portions as you proceed with the diet but at least you will have what you need and save yourself some trips to the store.

3. Wash, dry, cut and store all of the foods that you need, that way you have them conveniently prepared when you need them. This will make a new diet seem less tedious.

One necessary kitchen tool that you will need aside from the actual foods is a juicer. You will need a juicer as soon as you start the Sirtfood diet. Juicers are everywhere so they are quite easy to find, but the quality ranges greatly however. This is where price, function, and convenience comes into play. You could go to a popular department store, or you can find them online. Once you know what you are going after, you can shop around.

The quality of the juicer will also determine the nutritional quality and sometimes the taste of your juice, which we will explain a bit later. Just know that buying a cheap juicer may seem like a good idea now, but if you decide to upgrade later you will have spent more money, and twice. If you buy a good juicer, think of it like an investment into your health. Many people have spent money for a gym membership that went unused for quadruple the cost of one juicer. A juicer won't go to waste.

So, since not all juicers are alike, let us list a few of the features that you want to look for.

Centrifugal juicers:

Centrifugal juicers do just that, they use centrifugal force to spin the food most like vegetables like carrots, cucumbers, or kale leaves at high speeds to the side walls, where there are blades. The food is pushed through a sieve and then you have your juice. You have to drink this rather quickly, as you will lose nutrients the longer it is exposed to air which it already has done as it was spinning, and it oxidizes, as well as a bit of heat from the friction which creates a loss of nutrients and enzymes. This is the whole reason you are juicing, so this point is quite important. You are also left with a lot of solid but very wet pulp as a byproduct, which also means there was a lot of fibrous parts of the plants that the juicer couldn't handle. This is also a missed opportunity for more nutrients. You will also get a lot of warmish foam at the top, which some people do not like. It is quick and it is easy however, and it is usually the cheapest of the juicer types. If you must it is better than not having one at all, but if you can make an investment, you will reap your rewards later.

Masticating juicers:

Masticating juicers also do what they say they are. They masticate or chew the food, albeit more slowly than the other type, by pulling it through gears which extract the juice. The machine pushes the pulp out. You would have less pulp with this machine afterwards. There is also less oxidation, and thus, more nutrients. They also can handle other types of foods which varies by make and model, but that is something you should consider. You will get some foam with this as well, but not as much. These are more expensive, and again, should be looked at as you would an investment that you would not use and toss away. If you want it to last, and you want to get the most from your juicing and take it seriously, you will want to spend a bit more money and get what you really need.

Twin-gear/triturating juicers:

These geared juicers have gears that grind together with millimeters of space left between, to really tear open foods and grind the plants with only a very dry pulp that is left. These are the most nutrient-efficient juicers on the market. They leave virtually no foam and they are nutrient-dense as they are not disturbing the inner plant cells with oxidation. You usually can tell in the look of color and taste richer than other juices. You can use different attachments to make different foods with most brands as well, so they are versatile. These are the highest pricing of most of the juicers in general, and there are also brand variations as with the others.

Note: If all else fails, in a pinch and with a blender you could get away with a very poor quality juice by blending the foods, and using a fine mesh to filter the juice that is left. The only problem is that you would be getting a fraction of the nutrients, and also probably a spike in sugar, as very little fiber will be in the juice to help slow down the natural sugar absorption. Use caution.

Some of the juice recipes call for things that are too soft for most juices, such as if you were to use watermelon. You cannot juice a watermelon, so you should definitely use a blender. A good blender that can work quickly, and has a good strong motor will be a good investment as well.

Citrus Juicers

There are also juicers specifically for citrus fruits. These can range from hand held, col-press juicers, to small electric or automatic cold-press juicers. They too vary in quality and price,

It will help engage your more in the process and journey you are about to take! Storing Juices

The most nutrition from them immediately, you should drink them right away. If needed you can pre-juice, and put them in glass jelly, Mason jars. The wide mouth variety with the plastic lids is good, airtight and non-corrosive.

You can chill your drinks for the day, by resting them on ice packs in an insulated lunch tote or cooler. In extreme cases, you could juice one to three days of them it is recommended at the maximum for optimal freshness, although you could push it further out.

You may also find something to keep the juice chilled even while you are drinking at home. You can put a jar in the refrigerator just before prepping, and after you juice, pour it into one. You can make it a regular ritual of sorts. Have "your glass" that you get ready every day. If you prefer straws, you can even buy yourself a nice, reusable glass straw. None of these things are necessary for the diet, but any juice just tastes so much better when it is not from plastic.

Here are some other tips to help you get started:

Drink your juices as the earlier meals in the day if it helps you. It is a great way to start your day for three reasons.

- It will give you energy for breakfast and for lunch especially. By not having to digest heavy foods, your body saves time and energy usually spent on moving things around to go through all the laborious motions. You will be guaranteed to feel lighter and more energetic this way. You can always change this pattern after the maintenance phase, but you may find that you want to keep that schedule.

- Having fruits and vegetables before starchy or cooked meals, no matter how healthy the ingredients, is the best way to go for your digestion. Fruits and vegetables digest more rapidly, and the breakdown into the compounds that we can use more readily. Think of it as having your salad before your dinner. It works in the same way. The heavier foods, grains, oils, meats, etc., take more time to digest. If you eat these first, they will slow things down and that is where you have a backup of food needing to be broken down. This is also when you may find yourself with indigestion.

- Juices, especially green juices contain phytochemicals that not only serve as anti-oxidants but they contribute to our energy and mood. You will notice that you feel much differently after drinking a green juice than you would if you had eggs and sausage. You may want to make a food diary and note things such as this!

Be prepared to adjust to having lighter breakfasts for a little while. Most often we fill up with high protein, carbohydrate, and high calorie meals early in the day. We may feel that we did not get enough to eat and that we are not full at first. Oddly as it sounds, we may even miss the action of chewing. Some people need to chew their food to feel like they have had a filling meal. It is something automatic that we do not think of. Some also will miss that crunch such as with toast. Just pay attention to this, and know this is normal, and that it will pass.

THE PHASES OF THE SIRT DIET

For every newbie, it is important to understand that the Sirtfood diet does not start with a single list of ingredients in your hands. Its implementation and adaptation are more than mere selective grocery shopping. Every diet can only work effectively when we allow our body to embrace the sudden shift and change in food intake. Similarly, the Sirtfood diet also comes with two phases of adaptation. If a dieter successfully goes through these phases, he can continue with the Sirtfood diet easily. There are mainly two phases of this diet which are then succeeded by a third phase in which you can decide how you want to continue the diet.

Phase One

The first seven days of this diet plan are characterized as Phase One. In this phase, a dieter must focus on calorie restriction and the intake of green juices. These seven days are crucial to initiate your weight loss and usually helps to lose up to seven pounds if the diet is followed properly. If you find yourself achieving this target that means that you are on the right track.

In the first three days of the first phase, a dieter must restrict this caloric intake to 1,000 calories only. While doing so, the dieter must also have green juice throughout the day, probably three times a day. Try to drink green juice per meal. The recipes given in the Guidelines are perfect to select from.

There are many meal options that can keep your caloric intake in check such as buckwheat noodles, seared tofu, some shrimp stir fry, or Sirtfood omelet.

Once the first three days of this diet has passed, you can increase your caloric intake to 1,500 calories per day. In these next four days, you can reduce the green juices to two times per side. And pair the juices with more Sirtuin-rich food in every meal.

1.Matcha Green Juice

Preparation time: 10 minutes

Cooking Time: 10 minutes

Servings: 2

INGREDIENTS

- 5 ounces fresh kale
- 2 ounces fresh arugula
- ¼ cup fresh parsley
- 4 celery stalks
- 1 green apple, cored and chopped
- 1 1-inch piece fresh ginger, peeled
- 1 lemon, peeled
  - ½ teaspoon matcha green tea

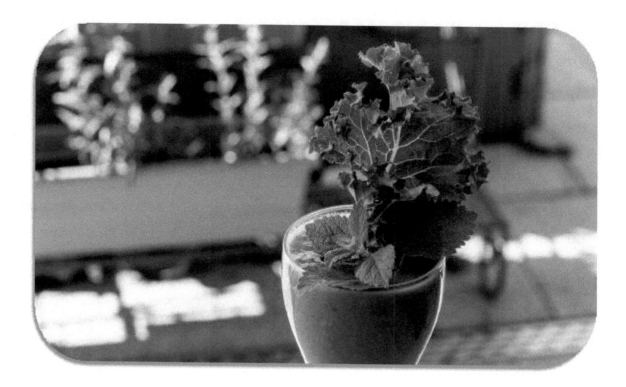

DIRECTIONS

1. Add all ingredients into a juicer and extract the juice according to the manufacturer's method.

2. Pour into 2 glasses and serve immediately.

NUTRITION: Calories 113 Total Fat 0.6 g Saturated Fat 0.1 g Cholesterol 0 mg Sodium 71 mg Total Carbs 26.71 g Fiber 5.3 g Sugar 12.9 g Protein 3.8 g

2.Celery Juice

Preparation time: 10 minutes

Cooking Time: 10 minutes

Servings: 2

INGREDIENTS

- 8 celery stalks with leaves

- 2 tablespoons fresh ginger, peeled

- 1 lemon, peeled

- ½ cup filtered water

- Pinch of salt

DIRECTIONS

1. Blend all ingredients, pulse until well combined.

2. Strain the juice and transfer into 2 glasses.

3. Serve immediately

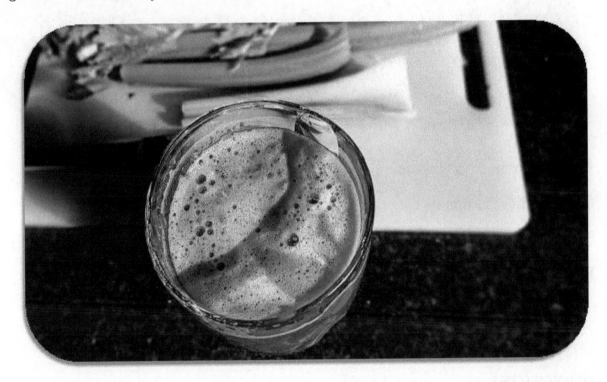

NUTRITION: Calories 32 Total Fat 0.5 g Saturated Fat 0.1 g Cholesterol 0 mg Sodium 134 mg Total Carbs 6.5 g Fiber 2 g Sugar 1.3 g Protein 1 g

3.Kale & Orange Juice

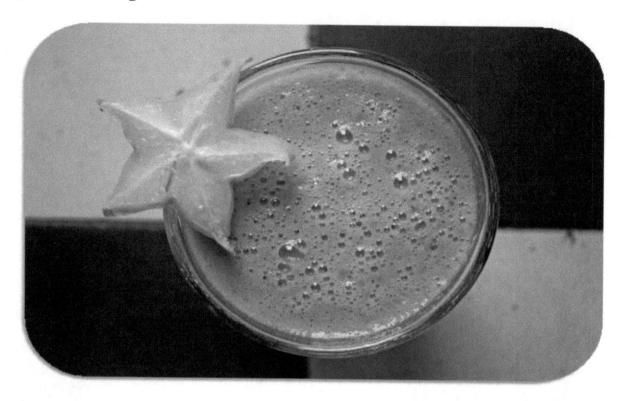

Preparation time: 10 minutes

Cooking Time: 10 minutes

Servings: 2

INGREDIENTS

- 5 large oranges, peeled and sectioned
- 2 bunches fresh kale

DIRECTIONS

1. Add all ingredients into a juicer and extract the juice according to the manufacturer's method.

2. Pour into 2 glasses and serve immediately.

NUTRITION: Calories 315 Total Fat 0.6 g Saturated Fat 0.1 g Cholesterol 0 mg Sodium 87 mg Total Carbs 75.1 g Fiber 14 g Sugar 4.3 g Protein 10.3 g

4.Apple & Cucumber Juice

Preparation time: 10 minutes

Cooking Time: 10 minutes

Servings: 2

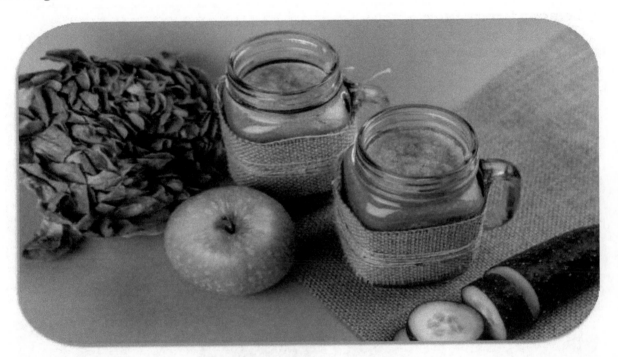

INGREDIENTS

- 3 large apples, cored and sliced
- 2 large cucumbers, sliced
- 4 celery stalks
- 1 1-inch piece fresh ginger, peeled
- 1 lemon, peeled

DIRECTIONS

1. Add all ingredients into a juicer and extract the juice according to the manufacturer's method.

2. Pour into 2 glasses and serve immediately.

NUTRITION: Calories 230 Total Fat 1.1 g Saturated Fat 0.1 g Cholesterol 0 mg Sodium 37 mg Total Carbs 59.5 g Fiber 10.5 g Sugar 40.5 g Protein 3.3 g

5.Lemony Green Juice

Preparation time: 10 minutes

Cooking Time: 10 minutes

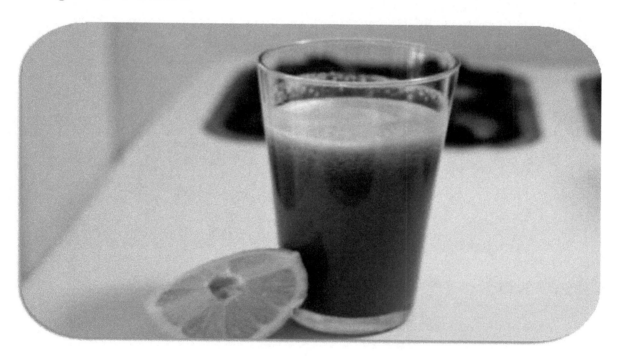

Servings: 2

INGREDIENTS

- 2 large green apples, cored and sliced

- 4 cups fresh kale leaves

- 4 tablespoons fresh parsley leaves

- 1 tablespoon fresh ginger, peeled

- 1 lemon, peeled

- ½ cup filtered water

- Pinch of salt

DIRECTIONS

1. Blend all ingredients.

2. Strain the juice and transfer into 2 glasses.

3. Serve immediately.

NUTRITION: Calories 196 Total Fat 0.6 g Saturated Fat 0.1 g Cholesterol 0 mg Sodium 143 mg Total Carbs 47.9g Fiber 8.2 g Sugar 23.5 g Protein 5.2 g

6. Kale Scramble

Preparation time: 10 minutes

Cooking time: 6 minutes

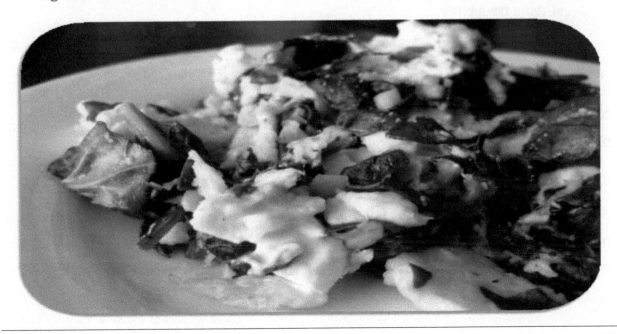

Servings: 3

INGREDIENTS

- 4 eggs

- 1/8 teaspoon ground turmeric

- Salt and ground black pepper, to taste

- 1 tablespoon water

- 2 teaspoons olive oil

- 1 cup fresh kale, tough ribs removed and chopped

DIRECTIONS

1. In a bowl, add the eggs, turmeric, salt, black pepper, and water and with a whisk, beat until foamy.

2. In a wok, heat the oil over medium heat.

3. Add the egg mixture and stir to combine.

4. Immediately, reduce the heat to medium-low and cook for about 1–2 minutes, stirring frequently.

5. Stir in the kale and cook for about 3–4 minutes, stirring frequently.

6. Remove from the heat and serve immediately.

NUTRITION: Calories 183 Total Fat 13.4 g Saturated Fat 3.4 g Cholesterol 327 mg Sodium 216 mg Total Carbs 4.3 g Fiber 0.5 g Sugar 0.7 g Protein 12.1 g

Phase Two

After the first week of the Sirtfood diet, then starts phase two. This phase is more about the maintenance of the diet, as the first week enables the body to embrace the change and start working according to the new diet. This phase enables the body to continue working towards the weight loss objective slowly and steadily. Therefore, the duration of this phase is almost two weeks.

So how is this phase different from the phase one? In this phase, there is no restriction on the caloric intake, as long as the food is rich in sirtuins and you are taking it three times a day, it is good to go. Instead of having the green juice two or three times a day, the dieter can have juice one time a day, and that will be enough to achieve steady weight loss. You can have the juice after any meal, in the morning or in the evening.

After the Diet Phase

With the end of phase two comes the time which is most crucial, and that is the after-diet phase. If you haven't achieved your weight loss target by the end of phase two, then you can restart the phases all over again. Or even when you have achieved the goals but still want to lose more weight, then you can again give it a try.

Instead of following phases one and two over and over again, you can also continue having good quality Sirtfood meals in this after-diet phase. Simply continue the eating practices of phase two, have a diet rich in sirtuin, and do have green juices whenever possible.

1. Apple & Celery Juice

Preparation time: 10 minutes

Cooking Time: 10 minutes

Servings: 2

INGREDIENTS

- 4 large green apples, cored and sliced

- 4 celery stalks

- 1 lemon, peeled

DIRECTIONS

1. Add all ingredients into a juicer and extract the juice according to the manufacturer's method.

2. Pour into 2 glasses and serve immediately.

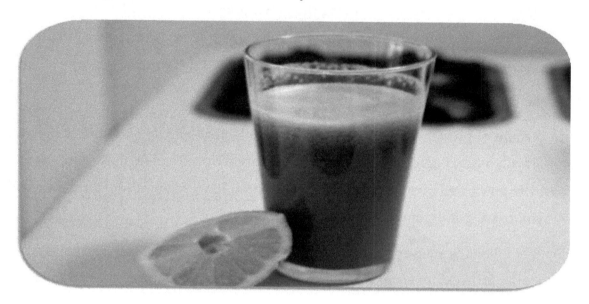

NUTRITION: Calories 240 Total Fat 0.9 g Saturated Fat 0 g Cholesterol 0 mg Sodium 31 mg Total Carbs 63.3 g Fiber 11.6 g Sugar 47.1 g Protein 1.5 g

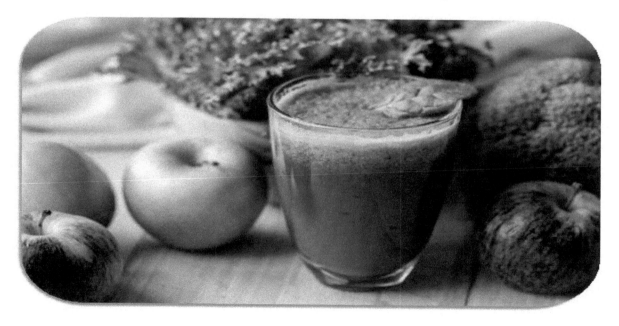

2.Broccoli, Apple, & Orange Juice

Preparation time: 10 minutes

Cooking Time: 10 minutes

Servings: 2

INGREDIENTS

- 2 broccoli stalks, chopped
- 2 large green apples, cored and sliced
- 3 large oranges, peeled and sectioned
- 4 tablespoons fresh parsley

DIRECTIONS

1. Add all ingredients into a juicer and extract the juice according to the manufacturer's method.
2. Pour into 2 glasses and serve immediately.

NUTRITION: Calories 254 Total Fat 0.8 g Saturated Fat 0.1 g Cholesterol 0 mg Sodium 11 mg Total Carbs 64.7 g Fiber 12.7 g Sugar 49.3 g Protein 3.8 g

3.Green Fruit Juice

Preparation time: 10 minutes

Cooking Time: 10 minutes

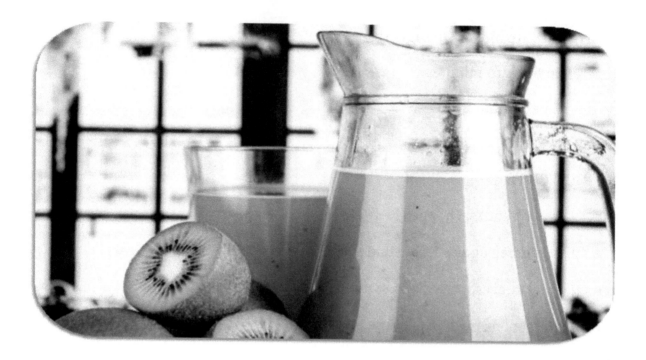

Servings: 2

INGREDIENTS

- 3 large kiwis, peeled and chopped

- 3 large green apples, cored and sliced

- 2 cups seedless green grapes

- 2 teaspoons fresh lime juice

DIRECTIONS

1. Add all ingredients into a juicer and extract the juice according to the manufacturer's method.

2. Pour into 2 glasses and serve immediately.

NUTRITION: Calories 304 Total Fat 2.2 g Saturated Fat 0 g Cholesterol 0 mg Sodium 6 mg Total Carbs 79 g Fiber 12.5 g Sugar 60.1 g Protein 6.2 g

4. Food plan of the first 7 days

Day 1

Breakfast: Matcha Green Juice

Lunch: Chicken, Kale, & Carrot Salad

Dinner: Lentils & greens Soup

Day 2

Breakfast: Kale Scramble

Lunch: Salmon Burgers

Dinner: Tofu & Broccoli Curry

Day 3

Breakfast: Blueberry Muffins

Lunch: Bok Choy & Mushroom Stir Fry

Dinner: Lamb Chops with Kale

Day 4

Breakfast: Buckwheat Granola

Lunch: Arugula, Strawberry, & Orange Salad

Dinner: Shrimp with Kale

Day 5

Breakfast: Broccoli, Apple, & Orange Juice

Lunch: Arugula & Berries Salad

Dinner: Chicken & Veggies with Buckwheat Noodles

Day 6

Breakfast: Matcha Pancakes

Lunch: Chickpeas with Swiss chard

Dinner: Beef & Kale Salad

Day 7

Breakfast: Chocolate Waffles

Lunch: Rocket & Orange Salad

Dinner: Prawns with Asparagus

QUICK AND EASY RECIPES FOR LUNCH

1.King Prawn Stir-fry & Soba

Preparation Time: 15 minutes

Cooking Time: 20 mutes

Servings: 3-4 servings

INGREDIENTS

- 150g shelled raw king prawns, deveined

- 2 tsp. tamari

- 2 tsp. extra virgin olive oil

- 75 soba

- 1 garlic clove, finely chopped

- 1 bird's eye chili, finely chopped

- 1 tsp. finely chopped fresh ginger

- 20g red onions, sliced

- 40g celery, trimmed and sliced

- 75g green beans, chopped

- 50g kale, roughly chopped

- 100ml chicken stock

DIRECTIONS

1. Warm a skillet over a high heat, and then fry for the pawns in 1 tsp. of the tamari and 1 tsp. of olive oil. Transfer the contents of the skillet to a plate, and then wipe the skillet with kitchen towel to remove the lingering sauce.

2. Boil water and cook the soba for 8 minutes, or according to packet instructions. Drain and set aside for later. Using the remaining 1 tsp. olive oil, fry the remaining ingredients for 3-4 minutes. Make the stock boil, simmering until the vegetables are tender but still have bite.

3. Add the lovage, noodles and prawn into the skillet, stir, bring back to the boil and then serve.

NUTRITION: 192 calories

2.Miso Caramelized Tofu

Preparation Time: 10 minutes

Cooking Time: 25

Servings: 3

INGREDIENTS

- 1 tbsp mirin

- 20g miso paste

- 1 * 150g firm tofu

- 40g celery, trimmed

- 35g red onion

- 120g courgette

- 1 bird's eye chili

- 1 garlic clove, finely chopped

- 1 tsp. finely chopped fresh ginger

- 50g kale, chopped

- 2 tsp. sesame seeds

- 35g buckwheat

- 1 tsp. ground turmeric

- 2 tsp. extra virgin olive oil

- 1 tsp. tamari or soy sauce

DIRECTIONS

1. Pre-heat your over to 200C or gas mark 6. Cover a tray with baking parchment.

2. Combine the mirin and miso together. Dice the tofu and coat it in the mirin-miso mixture in a resalable plastic bag. Set aside to marinate.

3. Chop the vegetables except for the kale at a diagonal angle to produce long slices. Using a steamer, cook for the kale for 5 minutes and set aside.

4. Disperse the tofu across the lined tray and garnish with sesame seeds. Roast for 20 minutes, or until caramelized.

5. Rinse the buckwheat using running water and a sieve. Add to a pan of boiling water alongside turmeric and cook the buckwheat according to the packet instructions.

6. Heat the oil in a skillet over high heat. Toss in the vegetables, herbs and spices then fry for 2-3 minutes. Reduce to a medium heat and fry for a further 5 minutes or until cooked but still crunchy.

NUTRITION: 192 calories

3.Sirtfood Cauliflower Couscous & Turkey Steak

Preparation Time: 10 minutes

Cooking Time: 15 minutes

Servings: 2

INGREDIENTS

- 150g cauliflower, roughly chopped
- 1 garlic clove, finely chopped
- 40g red onion, finely chopped
- 1 bird's eye chili, finely chopped
- 1 tsp. finely chopped fresh ginger
- 2 tbsp extra virgin olive oil
- 2 tsp. ground turmeric
- 30g sun dried tomatoes, finely chopped
- 10g parsley
- 150g turkey steak
- 1 tsp. dried sage
- Juice of ½ lemon
- 1 tbsp capers

DIRECTIONS

1. Disintegrate the cauliflower using a food processor. Blend in 1-2 pulses until the cauliflower has a breadcrumb-like consistency.

2. In a skillet, fry garlic, chili, ginger and red onion in 1 tsp. olive oil for 2-3 minutes.

Throw in the turmeric and cauliflower then cook for another 1-2 minutes. Remove from heat and add the tomatoes and roughly half the parsley.

3. Garnish the turkey steak with sage and dress with oil. In a skillet, over medium heat, fry the turkey steak for 5 minutes, turning occasionally. Once the steak is cooked add lemon juice, capers and a dash of water. Stir and serve with the couscous.

NUTRITION: 231 Calories

4.Mushroom & Tofu Scramble

Preparation Time: 10 minutes

Cooking Time: 10 minutes

Servings: 1

INGREDIENTS

- 100g tofu, extra firm

- 1 tsp. ground turmeric

- 1 tsp. mild curry powder

- 20g kale, roughly chopped

- 1 tsp. extra virgin olive oil

- 20g red onion, thinly sliced

- 50g mushrooms, thinly sliced

- 5g parsley, finely chopped

DIRECTIONS

1. Place 2 sheets of kitchen towel under and on-top of the tofu, then rest a considerable weight such as saucepan onto the tofu, to ensure it drains off the liquid.

2. Combine the curry powder, turmeric and 1-2 tsp. of water to form a paste. Using a steamer cook kale for 3-4 minutes.

3. In a skillet, warm oil over a medium heat. Add the chili, mushrooms and onion, cooking for several minutes or until brown and tender.

4. Break the tofu in to small pieces and toss in the skillet. Coat with the spice paste and stir, ensuring everything becomes evenly coated. Cook for up to 5 minutes, or until the tofu has browned then add the kale and fry for 2 more minutes. Garnish with parsley before serving.

NUTRITION: 232 calories

5.Prawn & Chili Pak Choi

Preparation Time: 10 minutes

Cooking Time: 10 minutes

Servings: 1

INGREDIENTS

- 75g brown rice
- 1 pak choi
- 60ml chicken stock
- 1 tbsp extra virgin olive oil
- 1 garlic clove, finely chopped
- 50g red onion, finely chopped
- ½ bird's eye chili, finely chopped
- 1 tsp. freshly grated ginger
- 125g shelled raw king prawns
- 1 tbsp soy sauce
- 1 tsp. five-spice

- 1 tbsp freshly chopped flat-leaf parsley

- A pinch of salt and pepper

DIRECTIONS

1. Bring a medium sized saucepan of water to the boil and cook the brown rice for 25-30 minutes, or until softened.

2. Tear the pak choi into pieces. Warm the chicken stock in a skillet over medium heat and toss in the pak choi, cooking until the pak choi has slightly wilted.

3. In another skillet, warm olive oil over high heat. Toss in the ginger, chili, red onions and garlic frying for 2-3 minutes.

4. Throw in the pawns, five-spice and soy sauce and cook for 6-8 minutes, or until the cooked throughout. Drain the brown rice and add to the skillet, stirring and cooking for 2-3 minutes. Add the pak choi, garnish with parsley and serve.

NUTRITION: 193 calories

6.Sirtfood Granola

Preparation Time: 10 minutes

Cooking Time: 25 minutes

Servings: 12

INGREDIENTS

- 200g oats

- 250g buckwheat flakes

- 100g walnuts, chopped

- 100g almonds, chopped

- 100g dried strawberries

- 1 ½ tsp. ground ginger

- 1 ½ tsp. ground cinnamon

- 120mls olive oil

- 2 tbsp honey

DIRECTIONS

1. Preheat your oven to 150C. Line a tray with baking parchment.

2. Stir together walnuts, almonds, buckwheat flakes and oats with ginger and cinnamon. In a large pan, warm olive oil and honey, heating until the honey has dissolved.

3. Pour the honey-oil over the other ingredients, stirring to ensuring an even coating. Separate the granola evenly over the lined baking tray and roast for 50 minutes, or until golden.

4. Once cooled add the berries and store in an airtight container. Eat dry or with milk and yogurt. It stays fresh for up to 1 week.

NUTRITION: 231 calories

7.Tomato Frittata

Preparation Time: 10 minutes

Cooking Time: 15 minutes

Servings: 2

INGREDIENTS

- 50g cheddar cheese, grated

- 75g kalamata olives, pitted and halved

- 8 cherry tomatoes, halved

- 4 large eggs

- 1 tbsp fresh parsley, chopped

- 1 tbsp fresh basil, chopped
- 1 tbsp olive oil

DIRECTIONS

1. Whisk the eggs in a mixing bowl. Toss in the parsley, basil, olives, tomatoes and cheese, stirring thoroughly.

2. Heat the olive oil over high heat. Pour in the frittata mixture and cook for 5-10 minutes, or set. Remove the skillet from the hob and place under the grill for 5 minutes, or until firm and set. Divide into portions and serve immediately.

NUTRITION: 231 calories

8.Horseradish Flaked Salmon Fillet & Kale

Preparation Time: 10 minutes

Cooking Time: 15 minutes

Servings: 2

INGREDIENTS

- 200g skinless, boneless salmon fillet
- 50g green beans
- 75g kale
- 1 tbsp extra virgin olive oil
- ½ garlic clove, crushed
- 50g red onion, chopped
- 1 tbsp fresh chives, chopped
- 1 tbsp freshly chopped flat-leaf parsley
- 1 tbsp low fat crème fraiche

- 1tbsp horseradish sauce

- Juice of ¼ lemon

- A pinch of salt and pepper

DIRECTIONS

1. Preheat the grill.

2. Sprinkle a salmon fillet with salt and pepper. Place under the grill for 10-15 minutes. Flake and set aside.

3. Using a steamer, cook the kale and green beans for 10 minutes.

4. In a skillet, warm the oil over a high heat. Add garlic and red onion and fry for 2-3 minutes. Toss in the kale and beans, and then cook for 1-2 minutes more.

5. Mix the chives, parsley, crème fraiche, horseradish, lemon juice and flaked salmon.

6. Serve the kale and beans topped with the dressed flaked salmon.

NUTRITION: 221 calories

9.Indulgent Yoghurt

Preparation Time: 10 minutes

Cooking Time: 15 minutes

Servings: 3

INGREDIENTS

- 125 mixed berries

- 150g Greek yoghurt

- 25 walnuts, chopped

- 10g dark chocolate at least 85% cocoa solids, grated

DIRECTIONS

1. Toss the mixed berries into a serving bowl. Cover with yoghurt and top with chocolate and walnuts. Voila!

NUTRITION: 231 calories

10.Tuna Salad

Preparation Time: 5 minutes

Cooking Time: 5 minutes

Servings: 1

INGREDIENTS

- 100g red chicory

- 150g tuna flakes in brine, drained

- 100g cucumber

- 25g rocket

- 6 kalamata olives, pitted

- 2 hard-boiled eggs, peeled and quartered

- 2 tomatoes, chopped

- 2 tbsp fresh parsley, chopped

- 1 red onion, chopped

- 1 celery stalk

- 1 tbsp capers

- 2 tbsp garlic vinaigrette

DIRECTIONS

1. Put the ingredients in a bowl and serve.

NUTRITION: 245 calories

11.Chicken & Bean Casserole

Preparation Time: 10 minutes

Cooking Time: 15 minutes

Servings: 2

INGREDIENTS

- 400g 14oz chopped tomatoes
- 400g 14oz tinned cannellini beans or haricot beans
- 8 chicken thighs, skin removed
- 2 carrots, peeled and finely chopped
- 2 red onions, chopped
- 4 sticks of celery
- 4 large mushrooms
- 2 red peppers bell peppers, de-seeded and chopped
- 1 clove of garlic
- 2 tablespoons soy sauce
- 1 tablespoon olive oil
- 1.75 liters 3 pints chicken stock broth

DIRECTION

1. Put and heat olive oil, add the garlic and onions and cook for 5 minutes.
2. Add in the chicken and cook for 5 minutes then add the carrots, cannellini beans, celery, red peppers bell peppers and mushrooms.
3. Pour in the stock broth soy sauce and tomatoes.

4. Bring it to the boil, reduce the heat and simmer for 45 minutes.

5. Serve with rice or new potatoes.

NUTRITION: 509 calories

---

12. Mussels in Red Wine Sauce

Preparation Time: 20 minutes

Cooking Time: 10 minutes

Servings: 2

INGREDIENTS

- 800g 2lb mussels

- 2 x 400g 14oz tins of chopped tomatoes

- 25g 1oz butter

- 1 tablespoon fresh chives, chopped

- 1 tablespoon fresh parsley, chopped

- 1 bird's-eye chili, finely chopped

- 4 cloves of garlic, crushed

- 400mls 14fl oz red wine

- Juice of 1 lemon

DIRECTION

1. Wash the mussels, remove their beards and set them aside.

2. Put butter in a saucepan. Add in the red wine.

3. Reduce the heat and add the parsley, chives, chili and garlic whilst stirring.

4. Add in the tomatoes, lemon juice and mussels.

5. Cover the saucepan and cook for 2-3.

6. Remove the saucepan from the heat and take out any mussels which haven't opened and discard them.

7. Serve and eat immediately.

NUTRITION: 364 calories

QUICK AND EASY RECIPES FOR BREAKFAST

13.Green Omelet

Preparation time: 10 minutes

Cooking Time: 10 minutes

Serving: 1

INGREDIENTS

- 2 large eggs, at room temperature

- 1 shallot, peeled and chopped

- Handful arugula

- 3 sprigs of parsley, chopped

- 1 tsp. extra virgin olive oil

- Salt and black pepper

DIRECTIONS

1. Beat eggs in a bowl then set aside. Sauté the shallot for 5 minutes with a bit of the oil, onlow-medium heat. Pour the eggs in the pans, stirring the mixture for just a second.

2. The eggs on a medium heat, and tip the pan just enough to let the loose egg run underneath after about one minute on the burner. Add the greens, herbs, and the

seasonings to the top side as it is still soft. TIP: You do not even have to flip it, as you can just cook the egg slowly egg as is well being careful as to not burn.

NUTRITION: 234 calories

14.Berry Oat Breakfast Cobbler

Preparation time: 10 minutes

Cooking Time: 10 minutes

Serving: 2

INGREDIENTS

- 2 cups of oats/flakes that are ready without cooking
- 1 cup of blackcurrants without the stems
- 1 teaspoon of honey or ¼ teaspoon of raw sugar
- ½ cup of water add more or less by testing the pan
- 1 cup of plain yogurt or soy or coconut

DIRECTIONS

1. Boil the berries, honey and water and then turn it down on low. Put in a glass container in a refrigerator until it is cool and set about 30 minutes or more

2. When ready to eat, scoop the berries on top of the oats and yogurt. Serve immediately.

NUTRITION: 234 calories

15.Pancakes with Apples and Blackcurrants

Preparation time: 10 minutes

Cooking Time: 10 minutes

Serving: 4

INGREDIENTS

- 2 apples, cut into small chunks

- 2 cups of quick cooking oats

- 1 cup flour of your choice

- 1 tsp. baking powder

- 2 tbsp. raw sugar, coconut sugar, or 2 tbsp. honey that is warm and easy to distribute

- 2 egg whites

- 1 ¼ cups of milk or soy/rice/coconut

- 2 tsp. extra virgin olive oil

- A dash of salt

For the berry topping:

- 1 cup blackcurrants, washed and stalks removed

- 3 tbsp. water may use less

- 2 tbsp. sugar see above for types

DIRECTIONS

1. Place the ingredients for the topping in a small pot simmer, stirring frequently for about 10 minutes until it cooks down and the juices are released.

2. Take the dry ingredients and mix in a bowl. After, add the apples and the milk a bit at a time, you may not use it all until it is a batter. Stiffly whisk the egg whites and then gently mix them into the pancake batter. Set aside in the refrigerator.

3. Pour a one quarter of the oil onto a flat pan or flat griddle, and when hot, pour some of the batter into it in a pancake shape. When the pancakes start to have golden brown edges and form air bubbles, they may be ready to be gently flipped.

4. Test to be sure the bottom can life away from the pan before actually flipping. Repeat for the next three pancakes. Top each pancake with the berries.

NUTRITION: 337 calories

16.Granola- the Sirt way

Preparation time: 10 minutes

Cooking Time: 10 minutes

Serving: 1

INGREDIENTS

- 1 cup buckwheat puffs

- 1 cup buckwheat flakes ready to eat type, but not whole buckwheat that needs to be cooked ½ cup coconut flakes

- ½ cup Medjool dates, without pits, chopped into smaller, bite-sized pieces

- 1 cup of cacao nibs or very dark chocolate chips

- 1/2 cup walnuts, chopped

- 1 cup strawberries, chopped and without stems 1 cup plain Greek, or coconut or soy yogurt.

DIRECTIONS

1. Mix, without yogurt and strawberry toppings.

2. You can store for up to a week. Store in an airtight container.

3. Add toppings even different berries or different yogurt.

4. You can even use the berry toppings as you will learn how to make from other recipes.

NUTRITION: 234 calories

17.Ginger Prawn Stir-Fry

Preparation time: 10 minutes

Cooking Time: 10 minutes

Serving: 1

INGREDIENTS

- 6 prawns or shrimp peeled and deveined
- ½ package of buckwheat noodles called Soba in Asian sections
- 5-6 leaves of kale, chopped
- 1 cup of green beans, chopped
- 5 g lovage or celery leaves
- 1 garlic clove, finely chopped
- 1 bird's eye chili, finely chopped
- 1 tsp. fresh ginger, finely chopped
- 2 stalks celery, chopped
- ½ small red onion, chopped
- 1 cup chicken stock or vegetable if you prefer
- 2 tbsp. soy sauce
- 2 tbsp. extra virgin olive oil

DIRECTIONS

1. Cook prawns in a bit of the oil and soy sauce until done and set aside about 10-15 minutes.

2. Boil the noodles according the instructions usually 6-8 minutes. Set aside.

3. Sauté the vegetables, then add the garlic, ginger, red onion, chili in a bit of oil until tender and crunchy, but not mushy. Add the prawns, and noodles, and simmer low about 5-10 minutes past that point.

NUTRITION: 234 calories

18. Chicken with Mole Salad

Preparation time: 10 minutes

Cooking Time: 10 minutes

Serving: 2

INGREDIENTS

- 1 skinned chicken breast
- 2 cups spinach, washed, dried and torn in halves
- 2 celery stalks, chopped or sliced thinly
- ½ cup arugula
- ½ small red onion, diced
- 2 Medjool pitted dates, chopped
- 1 tbsp. of dark chocolate powder
- 1 tbsp. extra virgin olive oil
- 2 tbsp. water
- 5 sprigs of parsley, chopped
- Dash of salt

DIRECTIONS

1. In a food processor, blend the dates, chocolate powder, oil and water, and salt. Add

the chili and process further. Rub this paste onto the chicken breast, and set it aside, in the refrigerator.

2. Prepare other salad mixings, the vegetables and herbs in a bowl and toss.

3. Cook the chicken in a dash of oil in a pan, until done, about 10-15 minutes over a medium burner.

4. When done, let cool and lay over the salad bed and serve.

NUTRITION: 23 calories

19.Strawberry Fields Salad

Preparation time: 10 minutes

Cooking Time: 10 minutes

Serving: 1

INGREDIENTS

- ½ cup cooked buckwheat
- 1 avocado, pitted, sliced and scooped
- 1 small tomato, quartered
- 2 Medjool dates, pitted
- 5 walnuts, chopped coarsely
- 20 g red onion
- 1 tbsp. capers
- 1 cup arugula
- 1 cup spinach
- 3 sprigs parsley, chopped
- 6 strawberries, sliced

- 1 tbsp. extra virgin olive oil

- ½ lemon, juiced

- 1 tbsp. ground turmeric

DIRECTION

1. Use room temperature buckwheat, or serve warm if preferred. Wash, dry and chop ingredients above, finish with the lemon and olive oil and turmeric as a dressing.

2. Add the buckwheat then the strawberries to the top of the salad.

NUTRITION: 231 calories

QUICK AND EASY RECIPES FOR SNACKS

20.Lemon Tofu Cheesecake

Preparation Time: minutes

Cooking Time: 40 minutes

Servings: 8

INGREDIENTS

- Silk tofu, drained – 24 ounces

- Almond butter – 1.5 tablespoons

- Date sugar – 1 cup

- Lemon zest – 1 teaspoon

- Sea salt .5 teaspoon

- Vanilla extract - .5 teaspoon

- Lemon juice - 2 tablespoons

- Cornstarch – 1.5 tablespoons

- Crust, 8-inch – 1 optional

DIRECTIONS

1. Preheat the oven to Fahrenheit three-hundred and fifty degrees. If you are preparing the lemon tofu cheesecake without a crust, I recommend preparing eight individual ramekins to divide the filling between. Otherwise, prepare an eight-inch crust of your choice.

2. Whisk together the lemon juice with the cornstarch to form a slurry.

3. In a food processor or blender combine the cornstarch slurry and remaining ingredients until fully combined, smooth, and creamy. You don't want any lumps.

4. Pour the lemon tofu cheesecake filling into the prepared crust or ramekins. If baking with the crust allow the cheesecake to cook until set, about thirty minutes. If you are using individual ramekins the cheesecake will only take fifteen to twenty-two minutes, depending on the size of the ramekins.

5. Allow the cheesecake to cool to room temperature, and then transfer it to the fridge until completely chilled through.

NUTRITION: Kilocalories per Individual Serving: 174

21. Blueberry Walnut Crisp

Preparation Time: minutes

Cooking Time: 35 minutes

Servings: 6

INGREDIENTS

- Walnuts, chopped - .25 cup

- Rolled oats - .5 cup

- Date sugar – 2 tablespoons

- Cinnamon, ground - .5 teaspoon

- Sea salt - .25 teaspoon

- Butter, cut into cubes – 2 tablespoons

- Blueberries – 4 cups

- Cornstarch – 1 tablespoon

- Date sugar – 2 tablespoons

- Lemon zest - .5 teaspoon

- Vanilla extract – 1 teaspoon

DIRECTIONS

1. Begin by preheating your oven to Fahrenheit three-hundred and fifty degrees and preparing six individual ramekins with non-stick cooking spray. Set the ramekins on a baking sheet to avoid spilling.

2. In a bowl toss together the blueberries with the cornstarch, date sugar, lemon zest, and vanilla. Once combined, divide the blueberries between the ramekins.

3. To make the crispy topping combine the remaining ingredients with a fork or pastry cutter. It will be crumbly. Top the blueberries in the ramekins with the crumble.

4. Set the baking sheet of ramekins in the oven and bake until golden-brown, about twenty-five to thirty minutes. Remove the blueberry walnut crisp from the oven and allow the crisps to cool slightly before serving.

NUTRITION: Kilocalories per Individual Serving: 214

22.Red Wine Poached Pears

Preparation Time: minutes

Cooking Time: 35 minutes

Servings: 6

INGREDIENTS

- Bosc pears – 6

- Cherries, pitted - .5 cup optional

- Red wine – 2 cups

- Orange juice - .5 cup

- Vanilla extract – 2 teaspoons

- Date sugar - .5 cup

- Cinnamon stick – 1

- Cloves, whole – 8

- Orange zest - .5 teaspoon

DIRECTIONS

1. Add all of your red wine poached pear ingredients, except for the Bosc pears, into a large Dutch oven. You need a pot large enough to fit all six whole hears. You want them to fit snugly so that the pears are fully covered in the liquid, but still have a slight wiggle room. But, remember, don't add the pears yet.

2. Allow the wine mixture to reach a simmer in the pot while stirring to dissolve the date sugar.

3. Wait until the poaching liquid has reached a simmer and then peel the pears. This will help avoid discoloration. Place the pears into the poaching liquid, arranging them so that they are submerged.

4. Allow the pears to continue simmering on medium-low for about twenty to twenty-five minutes. But, while the pears poach rearrange and rotate them every five minutes. Don't skip this, as it will ensure they poach evenly on all sides. You want to ensure even the tops of the pears are well poached.

5. Once the pears are done poaching, keep the pears upright in the wine mixture. Remove the pot from the heat of the stove, and allow both the pears and poaching liquid to cool down together.

6. While you can serve the poached pears once cooled to room temperature, I recommend first chilling them in the fridge.

7. When chilling the pears in the fridge, keep them stored in the liquid.

8. Once you are ready to serve the pears remove them from the liquid and set them on serving dishes. Meanwhile, add the poaching liquid into a saucepan and allow it to simmer to heat until it forms a slightly thickened syrup.

9. Pour the red wine syrup over the cold pears and serve.

NUTRITION: Kilocalories per Individual Serving: 266

23.Dark Chocolate Walnut No-Bake Cookies

Note: Not everyone has the time, energy, or oven needed to make traditional cookies. Plus, sometimes you might simply want to save on your electric bill. These cookies are just what you need in such times, as all you have to do is heat the ingredients together on the stove for a few minutes, no oven required!

Preparation Time: minutes

Cooking Time: 25 minutes

Servings: 24

INGREDIENTS

- Walnuts, chopped - .25 cups

- Coconut oil – 3 tablespoons

- Cocoa powder - .25 cup

- Dark chocolate chips - .5 cup

- Shredded coconut, unsweetened – 2 cups

- Almond butter - .5 cup

- Honey - .33 cup

- Vanilla extract – 1 teaspoon

- Sea salt - .25 teaspoon

DIRECTIONS

1. Prepare an aluminum baking sheet by covering it with kitchen parchment, wax coated paper, or a silicone mat.

2. Melt the coconut oil with the almond butter and honey over low heat in a saucepan. Once melted, stir in the remaining ingredients.

3. Use a tablespoon to scoop out portions of the chocolate walnut dough and roll each portion into a ball in your hands. Place the dark chocolate walnut no-bake cookie balls on the prepared baking sheet.

4. Freeze the cookies for ten minutes to set up. Enjoy immediately, or store the leftovers in a container in the freezer.

NUTRITION: Kilocalories per Individual Serving: 139

24.Quick Soft-Serve Cherry Sorbet

Preparation Time: minutes

Cooking Time: 5 minutes

Servings: 6

INGREDIENTS

- Cherries, frozen – 2 cups

- Bananas, frozen – 2

- Coconut milk, full-fat – 1 cup

DIRECTIONS

Add all of the sorbet ingredients to a blender, and combine until it is completely smooth without any chunks. It should be the consistency of soft-serve.

Enjoy the sorbet alone, or consider topping it with toasted coconut, roasted walnuts, or dark chocolate shavings.

NUTRITION:

Kilocalories per Individual Serving: 159

25.Honey-Roasted Plums with Ricotta

Note: These plums are a simple sweet treat, which allow fresh plums to really shine, especially when they are in-season. While they are best served with the ricotta, feel free to enjoy them with whipped cream, coconut cream, sorbet, ice cream, or even alone.

Preparation Time: minutes

Cooking Time: 20 minutes

Servings: 4

INGREDIENTS

- Plums, halved and pitted – 4

- Butter, melted – 1 tablespoon

- Honey – .25 cup

- Ricotta, part-skim, ideally fresh – 1 cup

DIRECTIONS

1. Begin by setting your oven to Fahrenheit four-hundred degrees and preparing a baking dish or skillet that can fit all eight plum halves. Add the melted butter into the dish.

2. Arrange your plum halves in the prepared dish, with the cut side facing upward. Drizzle the honey over the plums and bake until the plums are soft and release the juices, about fifteen minutes.

3. If you want to slightly char the plums, you can turn the broiler on for the last minute of baking.

4. Divide the roasted plums between serving dishes and top them with the ricotta. Serve while still warm.

NUTRITION: Kilocalories per Individual Serving: 206

---

26. No-Bake Triple Berry Mini Tarts

Preparation Time: minutes

Cooking Time: 20 minutes

Servings: 16

INGREDIENTS

- Frozen mixed berries, defrosted – 1 cup

- Honey - .5 cup

- Cacao butter, melted – 5 tablespoons

- Coconut cream - .33 cup

- Walnuts, raw – 2 cups

- Dates – 1 cup

DIRECTIONS

1. Combine walnuts in a food processor with the dates until it forms a crumbly mixture that can hold together when you press it. Scrape down the sides as needed.

2. Prepare a mini muffin tin for the crust, to make the mini tarts. Spray the pan with non-stick cooking spray.

3. Press the prepared crust into the mini muffin tin, forming mini tarts with crust pressed both on the bottom and on the sides of the muffin cups.

4. In a blender, mix the berries and other remaining ingredients until completely smooth. Divide the berry mixture between the crusts.

5. Place the filled muffin tin in the fridge and allow it to chill for six hours, or until set.

6. Use a kitchen knife to run around the edges of each tart to release them from the pan. Use a fork and take each tart out of the pan. Serve and enjoy!

NUTRITION: Kilocalories per Individual Serving: 190

---

27. Straverry Gurt

Preparation time: 20 Minutes

Cooking Time: 0 Minutes

Servings 2

INGREDIENTS

- 100g 3½ oz. strawberries

- 75g 3oz. frozen pitted cherries

- 1 tablespoon plain full-fat yogurt

- 175mls 6fl oz unsweetened soya milk

DIRECTIONS

1. Place all of the ingredients into a blender and process until smooth. Serve and enjoy.

NUTRITION: 132 calories per serving

---

28. Grape, Celery & Parsley Reviver

Preparation time: 10 Minutes

Cooking Time: 0 Minutes

Servings 2

INGREDIENTS

- 75g 3ozred grapes

- 3 sticks of celery

- 1 avocado, de-stoned and peeled

- 1 tablespoon fresh parsley

- ½ teaspoon matcha powder

DIRECTIONS

1. Place all of the ingredients into a blender with enough water to cover them and blitz until smooth and creamy.

2. Add crushed ice to make it even more refreshing.

NUTRITION: 334 calories per serving

29.Strawberry & Citrus Blend

Preparation time: 20 Minutes

Cooking Time: 0 Minutes

Servings 2

INGREDIENTS

- 75g 3ozstrawberries

- 1 apple, cored

- 1 orange, peeled

- ½ avocado, peeled and de-stoned

- ½ teaspoon matcha powder

- Juice of 1 lime

DIRECTIONS

1. Place all of the ingredients into a blender with enough water to cover them and process until smooth.

NUTRITION: 272 calories per serving

---

30. Watermelon Juice

Preparation time: 20 Minutes

Cooking Time: 0 Minutes

Servings 1

INGREDIENTS

- 20g of young kale leaves

- 250g of watermelon chunks

- 4 mint leaves

- ½ cucumber

DIRECTIONS

1. Remove the stalks from the kale and roughly chop it.

2. Peel the cucumber, if preferred, and then halve it and seed it.

3. Place all ingredients in a blender or juicer and process until you achieve a desired consistency. Serve immediately.

---

31. Green Tea Smoothie

Preparation time: 20 Minutes

Cooking Time: 0 Minutes

Servings 2

INGREDIENTS

- 2 teaspoons of honey
- 250 ml of milk
- 2 teaspoons of matcha green tea powder 6 ice cubes
- ½ teaspoon of vanilla bean paste not extractor a scrape of the seeds from vanilla pod
- 2 ripe bananas

DIRECTIONS

1. Place all the ingredients in a blender and run until you achieve a desired consistency.
2. Serve into two glasses and enjoy.

NUTRITION: 272 calories per serving

32. Berries Banana Smoothie

Preparation time: 10 Minutes

Cooking Time: 0 Minutes

Servings 2

INGREDIENTS

- ½ cup of coconut milk
- 1½ cups of mixed berries strawberries and blueberries)- could be frozen or fresh
- ¾ cup of water
- 4 ice cubes
- 1 tablespoon of molasses
- 1 banana

DIRECTIONS

1. Place all the ingredients in a blender and blend until smooth.

2. You can add water to the smoothie until you achieve your desired consistency then serve.

NUTRITION: 272 calories per serving

33.Mango & Rocket Arugula Smoothie

Preparation time: 10 Minutes

Cooking Time: 0 Minutes

Servings 2

INGREDIENTS

- 25g 1ozfresh rocket arugula

- 150g 5ozfresh mango, peeled, de-stoned and chopped

- 1 avocado, de-stoned and peeled

- ½ teaspoon matcha powder

- Juice of 1 lime

DIRECTIONS

1. Place all of the ingredients into a blender with enough water to cover them and process until smooth.

2. Add a few ice cubes and enjoy.

NUTRITION: 369 calories per serving

34.Grape and Melon Smoothie

Preparation time: 20 Minutes

Cooking Time: 0 Minutes

Servings 1

INGREDIENTS

- 100g of cantaloupe melon

- 100g of red seedless grapes

- 30g of young spinach leaves, stalks removed

- ½ cucumber

DIRECTIONS

1. Peel the cucumber, then cut it into half. Remove the seeds and chop it roughly.

2. Peel the cantaloupe, deseed it, and cut it into chunks.

3. Place all ingredients in a blender and blend until smooth.

NUTRITION:

369 calories per serving

35.Green Juice Recipe

Preparation time: 10 Minutes

Cooking Time: 0 Minutes

Servings 2

INGREDIENTS

- 1 large handful of rocket

- Two large handfuls of kale

- 1 very small handful of lovage leaves optional

- 2 or 3 large stalks of green celery including the leaves

- ½ medium green apple

- Juice of ½ lemon

- 1 very small handful of parsley

- ½ level teaspoon of matcha

DIRECTIONS

1. Mix the greens well and juice them to get about 50 ml of juice.

2. Juice the apple and the celery, and then peel the lemon and juice it by hand.

3. Pour a little of the juice in a glass, add matcha powder, and then stir vigorously. Once it has dissolved, pour it back on the juice, and stir it in. Add some water if the blend is a little too strong for you and serve.

NUTRITION: 369 calories per serving

HOW TO CALCULATE YOUR RDA

Prescribed Dietary Allowance: The RDA, the assessed measure of a supplement or calories every day considered fundamental for the upkeep of good wellbeing by the Food and Nutrition Board of the National Research Council/National Academy of Sciences. The RDA is refreshed intermittently to reflect new information. It is prominently called the Recommended Daily Allowance.

To decide your RDA for protein, increase your weight in pounds by 0.36. Or then again, attempt this online protein mini-computer. For instance, the RDA for a functioning, 45-year-elderly person weighing 175 lbs. is 64 g of protein daily. For a little 85-year-old inactive lady gauging 100 pounds, for her every day RDA of protein is 36 g.

"The RDA is the measurement of a supplement you have to meet your essential nourishing necessities," composed editorial manager Daniel Pendick on the Harvard Health Blog. "That is, it's the base sum you have to shield from becoming ill not the particular sum you should eat each day."

What amount of protein would you say you should eat each day?

A day by day protein admission of about 1.0-1.2 g/kg of body weight is advantageous for stable metabolic capacity, as indicated by look into bolstered by individuals from the Protein Summit 2.0. That is, about 10% to 35% of your complete calories in a day ought to be protein, they composed.

Protein Summit 2.0 was a gathering in October 2013 of more than 60 nourishment specialists and specialists from the United States and around the globe to decide the ideal protein requirements for human wellbeing. It's essential to take note of that the summit was supported by hamburger, egg, dairy, and pork industry gatherings. Yet, it brought about relevant reports that were freely distributed in an extraordinary enhancement to the American Journal of Clinical Nutrition.

A metabolically helpful protein consumption for an average grown-up ought to be 25-30 g for each supper, as per the Protein Summit's specialists. More established adults should eat somewhat more since they don't process protein just as more youthful grown-ups, they prescribed.

"Accordingly, unassumingly higher admissions of top-notch protein 1.0 g/kg to 1.5 g/kg every day, uniformly disseminated for the day, may maximally animate muscle protein blend, in this way adding to keeping up bulk in more established grown-ups," they composed.

What amount of protein do we get?

Things being what they are, are Americans getting enough or to an extreme protein? The average protein consumption for US grown-ups is 1.2 g/kg to 1.5 g/kg every day, or about 16% of their calories in protein, in light of 2003-2004 information from the NH National Health and NES Nutrition Examination Survey. Even though these qualities surpass the RDA, they are well underneath the Protein Summit's upper scope of 35% of calories for protein.

Protein consumption changes with age, sex, and activity level. For instance, youngsters ages 19-30 average 109 g of everyday protein while old ladies age 71 and more established get around 59 g for each day, as per the information.

What amount of nourishment is this?

It's hard for a great many people to picture in their minds how much protein is identical to, state, 0.8 g/kg of their body weight, or 25-30 g for each supper, or even 59 g for every day. Along these lines, here are a few models, as indicated by the US Department of Agriculture Food Composition Databases.

- ¼ cup almonds = 6 g protein

- 8 Oz skim milk = 8 g protein

- 2 hard-bubbled eggs = 13 g protein

- 1 cup stew with beans = 16 g protein

- 1/4 lbs. burger = 19 g protein

- 7 Oz plain low-fat Greek yoghurt = 20 g protein

- Ten chicken strips = 24 g protein

"It's additionally critical to consider the protein 'bundle' the fats, starches, nutrients, minerals, and different supplements that constantly join protein," Pendick composed. "Focus on protein sources low in soaked fat and prepared starches, and wealthy in numerous supplements." For instance, ten chicken tenders have 24 g of protein, yet they likewise accompany 26 g of fat. Two hard-bubbled eggs give 14 g protein however just 10.6 g fat, while bean stew has 15.7 g protein with just 9.6 g fat. Thus, bean stew gives less protein than chicken strips, however impressively less fat also. Similarly, as with any way to deal with better dietary wellbeing, teaching yourself just as your patients on these factors before settling on nourishment suggestions and decisions is constantly a smart thought.

Step by Step Procedure to calculate RDA:

To ascertain your prescribed dietary stipend, or RDA, for sugars, protein and fats, the principal thing you should do is decide your day by day caloric needs, given your body. When that is built up, you should determine your sugar, protein, and fat needs dependent on the suggested sums the body needs. As indicated by the ACE American Council on Exercise, your day by day diet should comprise of in any event 55 per cent starches, 15 per cent protein, and 30 per cent from fat. Eventually, these numbers can be somewhat balanced dependent on your individual needs.

Stage 1

Decide your day by day caloric needs dependent on your sex, age and movement level. As indicated by MyPyramid.gov, these components are expected to decide the total calories your body needs every day.

Stage 2

Duplicate your day by day caloric needs by the absolute suggested measure of sugars required every day. Since you're eating regimen ought to be roughly 55 per cent sugars, if your total caloric requirements for the day is 2400 calories, your condition will resemble this: 2400 X .55 = 1320. This implies 1320 calories you gobble every day ought to be comprised of starches.

Stage 3

Increase your day by day caloric needs by the all-out suggested measure of protein you need every day. Since you're eating regimen should comprise of around 15 per cent protein, your condition will resemble this: 2400 X .15 = 360. Out of your 2400 calories every day, 360 of them ought to be comprised of proteins.

Stage 4

Increase your day by day caloric needs by the full prescribed measure of fat you need every day. Since you're eating routine should comprise of around 30 per cent fat, your condition will resemble this: 2400 X.30 = 720. Out of your 2400 calories every day, 720 of them ought to be comprised of fats.

Stage 5

Take a gander at your dietary admission and ensure you are following what is suggested for you: 1320 calories from starches, 360 calories from protein, and 720 calories from fat.

How to set your meal plan:

Meal arranging is approaching the for supper question once for the entire week, rather than consistently, and afterwards looking for and preparing the fixings before cooking. We accept the most straightforward approach to move toward supper arranging is with three stages.

- Select your suppers and their plans, if necessary.

- Shop for ingredients.

- Set up those ingredients.

Start on a Friday: We're vast devotees of establishing this training throughout the end of the week, commencing the anticipating Friday, shopping on Saturday morning or night fewer individuals in the stores, and afterwards utilizing an hour or so on Sunday for supper prep.

Different Things Meal Planning Is Not

A primary selected cover with an entire month of suppers: Write it in your organizer, on a paper you adhere to the front of the refrigerator, in a Google Doc, or on a whiteboard you hang in the kitchen. Simply put it someplace you're going to see it.

Altogether home-cooked: We're huge, large fanatics of making arrangements for takeout, pizza night, and remains.

Only for groups of four: Meal arranging is for everybody. Be that as it may, there are various systems to utilize contingent upon the number of individuals you're getting ready for. In case you're flying performance, these tips for feast making arrangements for one are useful.

Costly: When progressed admirably, this training will set aside your cash. Guarantee!

A great deal of work: false. You do a touch of a real stir in advance, yet it's going great once you start to work your arrangement.

Firm: There's such a considerable amount of space for experimentation, speedy corrections, and customization in feast arranging. It's not unchangeable.

What Do You Need?

Presently, we're not requesting that you do profound soul looking, slightly self-evaluation. The least demanding approach to answering what you need the question is to consider why you're keen on dinner arranging by any means. From that point, we can focus on the best way to arrive. So for your thought, here are a couple of prompts.

- Is it exact to say that you are searching for assortment?

- To set aside cash?

- Eat better?

- Forestall nourishment squander?

- Safeguard your rational soundness?

- Or on the other hand to have a prepared response to the everyday question from your accomplice or children of what's for supper?

Dinner arranging is one of those circumstances where you can without a doubt have everything, except how about we do this gradually. Burnout is genuine, so in case you're a novice, pick only a few of the things that issue most and keep them in thought when you proceed onward to the following stage of choosing the plans our preferred part!

Pick Your Recipes Very Carefully

Picking your plans puts the way of thinking of dinner arranging and the reasons why you're doing it vigorously. We believe it's the most fundamental advance since it gets this entire procedure underway. Be that as it may, you shouldn't generally simply pick a lot of plans and trust in the best. Begin considering your supper plan, at any rate, three days before you need to give it back, so you have a couple of days to experience the full procedure of making a shopping rundown, shopping, and afterwards preparing. Here's how we prescribe you pick your plans.

Choose what number of suppers to get ready for and what they have to do.

Examine your schedule for the coming week and choose the number of evenings you need to make supper at home. Five evenings is the most well-known denominator, yet for specific individuals, three evenings is the sweet spot. At that point, you must sharpen in much further. On the evenings that you're cooking, what do those suppers need to do? For instance, in the evenings that your child has swim class, a 10-hour moderate cooker formula is a smart thought. On the off chance that it's merely you and your accomplice and she's working late, you may require something that you can likewise bring as tomorrow's lunch.

4 More Rules for Picking the Right Recipe

We have the subtleties on the best way to pick plans directly here, however here's its essence.

- Pick suppers that favor you with remains: They're the blessing that continues giving.

- Cook plans you know + one new formula: This is a genius move! Collect that ace rundown of plans you know by heart the ones you make without fail and realize your family cherishes. At that point include a couple of new ideas every week, except just on the off chance that you need.

- Pick plans dependent on regular fixings: This is another master move, and it begins with taking a gander at what you as of now have in your ice chest, more relaxed, and storeroom. Shopping your home kitchen can assist you with settling on plans and keep away from squandered nourishment. This is the cash sparing part of supper arranging in full impact.

SIRTUINS AND WEIGHT LOSS

Research conducted by Aidan Goggins and Glen Martin showed that 7 pounds of weight were lost on average in seven days on the Sirt food diet after taking note of muscle gain. Sirtuins' diet has not promised only weight loss; instead, good health as well. An increase in the level of body sirtuins has been proven to cause weight loss. The best way of increasing body lepton is still through fasting and exercise. Also, one of the best ways of enhancing body sirtuins is by consumption of sirtuin foods. All of the seas will affect body metabolism, which we will treat in the guide.

Furthermore, hypothalamic SIRT1 has been proven to help in weight loss. The hypothalamus is the central weight and energy balance controller. It modulates energy intake and energy consumption by neural inputs from the periphery as well as direct humor inputs, which senses the energy status of the body. An adipokine, lepton, is one of the factors that signal that sufficient energy is stored on the periphery. Lepton plasma levels are positive for adiposity, suppressing energy intake, and stimulating energy spending. A prolonged increase in the level of plasma lepton in obese can cause lepton resistance. Lepton resistance, in turn, can affect the hypothalamus from having access to lepton, which also reduces lepton signals transduction in the hypothalamic neurons. Reduced peripheral energy-sensing by lepton can lead to a positive energy balance and incremental weight gain and adiposity improvements, which further exacerbate lepton resistance. Lepton resistance causes an increase in adiposity, just like weight gain are all associated with ageing. Similar observations occur in central insulin resistance. The improvement of the action of hum oral factors in the hypothalamus can, therefore, prevent progressive weight gains, especially among middle-aged individuals. SIRT1 is a protein deacetylase, NAD+ dependent that has many substrates, such as transcription factors, histones, co-factors, and various enzymes. SIRT1 improves the sensitivity to lepton and insulin by decreasing the levels of several molecules that impair the transduction of lepton and insulin signals. The hypothalamic SIRT1 and NAD+ levels decrease with age. Increased in the level of SIRT1 has shown to improve kept in level in mice and so prevents age-related weight gain. By preventing the loss of age-dependent SIRT1 hypothalamus role, there will be a boost in the activity of hum oral factors in the hypothalamus and the central energy balance control.

Sirtuins, Fasting, and Metabolic Activities

SIRT1, just like other SIRTUINS family, is protein NAD+ dependent deacetylases that are associated with cellular metabolism. All sirtuins, including SIRT1 important for sensing energy status and in protection against metabolic stress. They coordinate cellular response towards Caloric Restrictions in an organism. SIRT1 diverse location and allows cells to easily sense changes in the level of energy anywhere in the mitochondria, nucleus, and cytoplasm. Associated with metabolic health through DE acetylation of several target proteins such as muscles, liver, endothelium, heart, and adipose tissue.

SIRT1, SIRT6, and SIRT7 are localized in the nucleus where they take part in the DE acetylation of customers to influence gene expression epigenetically. SIRT2 is located in the cytosol, while SIRT3, SIRT4, and SIRT5 are located in the mitochondria where they regulate metabolic enzyme activities as well as moderate oxidative stress.

SIRT1, as most studies with regards to metabolism, aid in mediating the physiological adaptation to diets. Several studies have shown the impact of sirtuins on Caloric Restriction. Sirtuins deacetylase non-histone proteins that define pathways involved during the metabolic adaptation when there are metabolic restrictions. Caloric Restriction, on the other hand, causes the induction of expression of SIRT1 in humans. Mutations that lead to loss of function in some sirtuins genes can lead to a reduction in the outputs of caloric restrictions. Therefore, sirtuins have the following metabolic functions:

Regulation in the liver

The Liver regulates the body glucose homeostasis. During fasting or caloric restriction, glucose level becomes low, resulting in a sudden shift in hepatic metabolism to glycogen breakdown and then to gluconeogenesis to maintain glucose supply as well as ketone body production to mediate the deficit in energy. Also, during caloric restriction or fasting, there is muscle activation and liver oxidation of fatty acids produced during lipolysis in white adipose tissue. For this switch to occur, there are several transcription factors involved to adapt to energy deprivation. SIRT1 intervenes during the metabolic switch to see the energy deficit.

At the initial stage of the fasting that is the post glycogen breakdown phase, there is the production of glucagon by the pancreatic alpha cells to active gluconeogenesis in the Liver through the cyclic amp response element-binding protein CREB, and CREB regulated transcription captivator 2 CRTC2, the captivator. Is the fasting gets prolonged, the effect is cancelled out and is being replaced by SIRT1 mediated CRTC2 deacetylase resulting in targeting of the captivator for ubiquitin/ proteasome-mediated destruction? SIRT1, on the other hand, initiates the next stage of gluconeogenesis through acetylation and activation of peroxisome proliferator-activated receptor captivator one alpha, which is the captivator necessary for forehead box O1. In addition to the ability of SIRT1 to support gluconeogenesis, captivator one alpha is required during the mitochondrial biogenesis necessary for the liver to accommodate the reduction in energy status. SIRT1 also activates fatty acid oxidation through DE acetylation and activation of the nuclear receptor to increase energy production. SIRT1, when involved in acetylation and repression of glycolytic enzymes such as phosphoglycerate mutate 1, can lead to shutting down of the production of energy through glycolysis. SIRT6, on the other hand, can be served as a co-repressor for hypoxia-inducible Factor 1 Alpha to repress glycolysis. Since SIRT6 can transcriptionally be induced by SIRT1, sirtuins can coordinate the duration of time for each fasting phase.

Aside from glucose homeostasis, the liver also overtakes in lipid and cholesterol homeostasis during fasting. When there are caloric restrictions, the synthesis of fat and cholesterol in the liver is turned off, while lipolysis in the white adipose tissue commences. The SIRT1, upon fasting, causes acetylation of steroid regulatory element-binding protein SREBP and targets the protein to destroy the ubiquitin-professor system. The result is that fat cholesterol synthesis will repress. During the regulation of cholesterol homeostasis, SIRT1 regulates ox sterol receptor, thereby, assisting the reversal of cholesterol transport from peripheral tissue through up regulation of the ox sterol receptor target gene ATP-binding cassette transporter A1 ABCA1.

Further modulation of the cholesterol regulatory loop can be achieved via bile acid receptor, that's necessary for the biosynthesis of cholesterol catabolic and bile acid pathways. SIRT6 also participates in the regulation of cholesterol levels by repressing the expression and post-translational cleavage of SREBP1/2, into the active form. Furthermore, in the circadian regulation of metabolism, SIRT1 participates through the regulation of cell circadian clock.

Mitochondrial SIRT3 is crucial in the oxidation of fatty acid in mitochondria. Fasting or caloric restrictions can result in up-regulation of activities and levels of SIRT3 to aid fatty acid oxidation through DE acetylation of long-chain specific acyl-CoA dehydrogenase. SIRT3 can also cause activation of ketogenesis and the urea cycle in the liver.

SIRT1 also Add it in the metabolic regulation in the muscle and white adipose tissue. Fasting causes an increase in the level of SIRT1, leading to DE acetylation of captivator one alpha, which in turn causes genes responsible for fat oxidation to get activated. The reduction in energy level also activates AMPK, which will activate the expression of captivator one alpha. The combined effects of the two processes will give rise to increased mitochondrial biogenesis together with fatty acid oxidation in the muscle.

Sirtuins and Exercise

The expression of sirtuin in the muscle is affected by physical exercise that controls changes in the cellular antioxidant system, mitochondrial biogenesis, and oxidative metabolism.

Skeletal muscles are not only involved in force and movement but also involved in endocrine activities by its ability to secrete cytokines and transcription factors into the bloodstream, thereby, controls the function of other organs. Furthermore, skeletal muscle is a metabolically active tissue that plays a vital role in maintaining the metabolism of the body. The skeletal muscle contains about 40% of the entire body weight. The insulin-stimulated uptake of glucose and the main energy-consuming lipid catabolism is mainly at this site. For the skeletal muscle, metabolic flexibility is essential to preserve physiological processes and metabolic homeostasis. It determines the ability to switch from glucose to lipid oxidation. Advances in the understanding of the molecular mechanisms underlying skeletal muscle activity are a therapeutic benefit. Sirtuins' roles have been widely investigated in the skeletal muscle concerning their role in controlling glucose and lipid metabolism, insulin functions and sensitivity as well as function, and mitochondrial biogenesis.

Cellular metabolic stress results from physical exercise, which affects the sirtuins. The most studies sirtuins with this respect are SIRT1 and SIRT3, SIRT1 localized in the nucleus while SIRT3, in the mitochondria. SIRT3 is more expressed in type I muscle fiber. A research conducted showed that mouse skeletal muscle SIRT3 reacted to the six weeks voluntary exercise dynamically to coordinate the downstream molecular response Palacios et al., 2009. The result also showed that exercise causes an increase in SIRT3 protein, CREB, captivator one alpha, and citrate synthesis activity.

The down regulation of CREB, AMP-activated protein kinase AMPK phosphorylation and the mRNA of PGC-1α are all symptoms of SIRT3 knockout. Showing that for SIRT3 to carry out the biological signals effectively, these key cellular molecules are essential. Palacios et al. discovered that SIRT3 responds to exercise dynamically to enhance muscular energy homeostasis through AMPK and PGC-1α. Voluntary exercise causes an increase in the SIRT3 content of skeletal muscle. Muscle Immobility can, therefore, lead to the down regulation of SIRT3.

Furthermore, SIRT1 protein content and PGC-1 in the muscle tends to increase with exercise. Beyond et al. 2012 reported that SIRT1 protein content, as well as PGC-1 in rat's muscle, increased after 36 weeks of treadmill training together with enhancement in antioxidant defenses. During exercise, there's an increase in demand for ATP, which in turn leads to increased NAD+ level and NAD+/NADH ratio. The result is an increase in the substrate for SIRT1 and SIRT3. SIRT3 is responsible for the increased ATP production as well as a reduction in protein synthesis in the mitochondria. The ATP produced activates and deacetylases tricarboxylic acid TCA enzymes, electron transport chain, and β-oxidation, which maximizes the availability of reducing equivalents for ATP production. SIRT1, on the other hand, responds to exercise by contributing towards mitochondrial biogenesis via independent mechanism and PGC1α-dependent.

In summary, strenuous exercises activate SIRT1, which enhances biogenesis and mitochondrial oxidative capacity. Then, having several sessions of exercise will activate both SIRT1 and also SIRT3, which in turn activate ATP production as well as the mitochondrial antioxidant function.

FOUR-WEEK PROGRAM

Let's be frank right from the beginning! You simply can't lose weight and boost your health overnight this can only happen in time. The Sirtfood diet is not a collection of recipes for magic potions. Although we encourage you to make the Sirtfood diet your default meal plan, the best way to find out if a diet is working is to monitor your results. In terms of weight loss, this can be so easily done, as you can check your weight on the scale on a daily basis more sophisticated scales can even show you're BMI, measure yourself around the waist, or check yourself in the mirror to notice any visible results. Obviously, medical results can't be monitored on a daily basis, as health improvements can only happen in time. There are plenty of health apps you can install on your smartphone to monitor different health indicators.

Therefore, you need a minimum period of time to test the Sirtfood diet, and the optimum time is four weeks. This period should be more than enough to show you the first signs of improvement when it comes to your health. So feel free to run a blood analysis after these four weeks, and monitor the triglyceride, cholesterol, and blood sugar level. There are a lot of indicators you can get from blood analysis, but there is no better proof that this diet really works.

Since the first week is the hardest one the seven-day meal plan, for the remaining four weeks of the program, we will try a more permissive program that includes a slight increase of calorie intake and three main meals per day. You will need to continue reading to find out more details about the maintenance phase. This is what comes after the first week, which is the intensive fat loss plan.

This program requires preparation to make the transition from your default diet to the Sirtfood one. Plenty of people are much stressed and just want to lose a lot of weight by constraining themselves to eat just a few ingredients. The Sirtfood diet is not like that, and it encourages you to try all sorts of ingredients. However, it helps you to combine them in such a way that reaps most of the weight loss and health benefits. The founders of this diet,

Aidan Goggins and Glen Matten, like to think that this is a diet of inclusion and no food is left behind. If you check the recipes included in this guidelines, you will see that these foods use a wide range of ingredients. You can have standard or vegan meals in order to enjoy diversity.

Sounds neat, right? You probably tried a lot of restrictive diets and perhaps even fasting. You either couldn't stick to a radical diet or had nasty side effects after following it was not good for your health, or you started to gain weight immediately after quitting it. Perhaps you are simply not satisfied with the results. This is where the Sirtfood diet can help you. So why not lose weight in a healthy and sustainable way? The cure to our medical problems caused by bad nutrition can be this interesting diet. Since this diet is very recent, perhaps you don't know anyone who has tried it before. How would you feel if you were envied for your physical shape and overall health? And when somebody asks you about your secret, you can mention the Sirtfood diet.

Well, this diet should deliver amazing results after just four weeks. This is why I encourage you to try for the four-week program at least. Therefore, if this diet works for you, why change it with a different one? Four weeks should be sufficient to find out whether the diet is appropriate for you or not.

MASTERS OF MUSCLES

One surprising result from our pilot trial that puzzled us was that the participants' muscle mass did not drop; instead, it rose by just over 1 pound on average. While it was common to see weight loss on the scales of 7 pounds, we saw something fascinating happening too. The injuries on the levels initially appeared more disappointing than this for almost two-thirds of our participants, though still very impressive, with a weight loss of just over 5 pounds. But when tests were done on body composition, we were astonished. In these participants, muscle mass was not only maintained; it had increased. The total muscle benefit for this category was almost 2 pounds, adding 7 pounds to what is called a "muscle gain-based weight loss."

This was totally unexpected and in stark contrast to what is typically the case for diets for weight loss, where people lose some fat but also lose muscle. For any diet which limits calories, it's the classic trade-off: you kiss good-bye muscle as well as fat.

What's good about maintaining Muscles?

So, what's that big deal? Do you know? Firstly, that means you're going to look much better. Stripping away weight while maintaining muscle leads to a healthy, toned, and competitive body that is more attractive. And more specifically, you should remain good looking. The skeletal muscle is the main factor that accounts for the daily energy output of our body, which ensures the more muscle that you have, the more calories that you use, even when you rest. This helps support further weight loss and increases the likelihood of long-term success. As we now learn, weight loss with typical diet results from both fat loss and muscle loss, and thereby we see a marked decline in the metabolic rate. This induces the body to regain weight once more regular eating habits are resumed. But you burn fatter with a minimal drop in metabolic rate by holding your muscle mass with Sirtfoods. This provides the perfect basis for weight-loss success over the long term.

In addition, muscle mass and function are predictors of well-being and healthy aging, and maintaining the muscle prevents the development of chronic diseases such as diabetes and osteoporosis, as well as keeping us mobile into older age. Importantly, it also seems to make us happy, with scientists believing that even the way sirtuins retain muscle has implications for stress-related disorders, including depression reduction.

All in all, weight loss when maintaining the body is a biggie and an even more desirable outcome. It's a unique feature of the Sirtfood Diet, and we need to get back to the sirtuins, so their substantial impact on the muscle to better understand why.

Sirtuins and Muscles Mass

In the body, there is a family of genes that function as guardians of our muscle and, when under stress, avoid its breakdown: the sirtuins. SIRT is a potent Muscle Breakdown Inhibitor. As long as SIRT is activated, even when we are fasting, muscle breakdown is prevented, and we continue to burn fat for fuel.

But SIRT's benefits aren't ending with preserving muscle mass. The sirtuins work to increase our skeletal muscle mass. We need to delve into the exciting world of stem cells and illustrate how that process functions. Our muscle comprises a particular type of stem cell, which is called a satellite cell that regulates its development and regeneration. Satellite cells just sit there quietly most of the time, but they are activated when a muscle gets damaged or stressed. By things like weight training, this is how our muscles grow stronger. SIRT is essential for activating satellite cells, and without its activity, muscles are significantly smaller because they no longer have the capacity to develop or regenerate properly.6 However, by increasing SIRT activity, we give a boost to our satellite cells, which encourages muscle growth and recovery.

Sirtfood versus Fasting

This leads to a big question: if activation of the sirtuin increases muscle mass, why do we lose muscle when we fast? Fasting also stimulates our sirtuin genes, after all. And therein is one of fasting's big pitfalls.

Stay with us as we dig into the mechanics of this. Not all skeletal muscles are created equal to each other. We have two main types, named type-1 and type-2, conveniently. Type-1 tissue is used for movements of longer duration, while the type-2 muscle is used for short bursts of more intense activity. And here's where it gets intriguing: fasting only increases SIRT activity in type-1 muscle fibers, not type-2, so type-1 muscle fiber size is maintained and even noticeably increases when we fast. Sadly, in complete contrast to what happens in type-1 fibers during fasting, SIRT rapidly decreases in type-2 fibers. This means that fat burning slows down, and muscle breaks down to provide fuel, instead.

But fasting for the muscles is a double-edged sword, with our type-2 fibers taking a hit. Type-2 fibers form the bulk of our concept of muscle. So even though our type-1 fiber mass is growing, with fasting, we still see a substantial overall loss of muscle. If we were able to stop the breakup, it would not only make us look aesthetically healthy but also help to promote more loss of weight. And the way to do this is to combat the decrease in SIRT in muscle fiber type-2 that is caused by fasting.

Researchers at Harvard Medical School tested this in an elegant mice study. They showed that the signals for muscle breakdown were switched off by stimulating SIRT activity in type-2 fibers during fasting, and no muscle loss occurred. The researchers then went to one step forward and checked the effects of increased SIRT behavior on the muscle while feeding the mice instead of fasted, and found it triggered a very rapid growth of the muscle. Within a week, muscle fibers with increased levels of SIRT activity showed an amazing weight gain of 20 percent.

These findings are very similar to the outcome of our Sirtfood Diet trial, though, in effect, our study has been milder. By increasing SIRT activity by eating a diet rich in sirtfoods, most participants had no muscle loss and for many, it was only a moderate fast, muscle mass that increased.

Keeping Muscles Young

And that is not just the thickness of the body. SIRT's prolific effects on the muscle extend to the way it works too. As the muscle ages, it loses the ability to activate SIRT. This makes it less sensitive to exercise benefits and more vulnerable to free radicals and inflammation destruction, resulting in what is known as oxidative stress. Gradually muscles wither, become softer, and fatigue faster. But if we can increase SIRT activation, we can stop the decline associated with aging.

Indeed, by activating SIRT to stop the loss of muscle mass and function we usually see with aging, we see multiple related health benefits, including the halting of bone loss and prevention of increased chronic systemic inflammation known as inflaming, as well as improvements in mobility and overall quality of life. So, interestingly, the latest research indicates that the higher the polyphenol level and thus sirtuin-activating nutrients in older people's diets, the higher the security they enjoy against deteriorating physical performance with age.

Don't be fooled into thinking that those incentives extend only to the elderly, far from that. By the age of twenty-five, the signs of aging will begin, and the muscle gradually erodes, with 10 percent loss of muscle around age forty although overall weight tends to increase and a loss of 40 percent by age seventy. Yet there is growing evidence that the activation of our sirtuin genes will inhibit and reverse all of this.

Loss of muscle, development, and function: sirtuin behavior plays a crucial role in all of this. Stack it up, and it's no surprise that sirtuins were identified as master regulators of muscle growth in a recent review in the prestigious medical journal Nature, with growing sirtuin activation cited as one of the promising new avenues for combating muscle loss, thereby increasing the quality of life, as well as reducing disease and death.

Looking at the powerful effects our sirtuin genes can have on the muscles, our pilot trial's shock results no longer seemed so shocking. We started to realize that driving weight loss when feeding our muscles was achievable through a diet rich in Sirtfood. But it's just the beginning.

- Amid weight loss, we found that people either retained or even gained muscle through the Sirtfood diet. This is because the sirtuins are chief muscle regulators.

- By activating sirtuins, muscle breakdown can be both prevented and muscle regeneration promoted.

- Triggering SIRT will help prevent the progressive muscle loss that we see with age.

- Activating your sirtuin genes will not only make you look leaner but will also help you stay healthier and function better as you age.

HOW SUPERFOODS PREVENT CANCER

A bowl brimming with splendid green steamed broccoli. You state either "Yum!" - Or "Where's the twofold cheeseburger?" But you realize the broccoli is beneficial for you, particularly without softened cheddar. The inquiry is, how acceptable? Furthermore, more to the point, can it - or any food - help forestall illness, for example, malignancy?

The appropriate response is yes - a few foods do show malignancy battling properties; however, nobody is yet ready to state some food can forestall or leave disease speechless.

In any case, an assortment of research recommends a general sound diet loaded up with brilliant products of the soil is the way to avoiding coronary illness, diabetes, and conceivably malignancy as well.

Actually, researchers find out about what not to eat - prepared meats, salty foods, sugary beverages, and enormous helpings of red meat - than which leafy foods to heap on your plate. Be that as it may, they do realize those foods matter.

A far reaching survey of thousands of concentrates on diet, physical movement, and weight led for the World Cancer Research Fund and the American Institute for Cancer Research highlighted the advantages of eating for the most part foods of plant starting point. Foods, for example, broccoli, berries, and garlic demonstrated the absolute most grounded connections to malignant growth anticipation.

They're low in calories and fat and force pressed with phytochemicals and cell reinforcements that may help diminish your malignant growth chance.

Cell reinforcements, Phytochemicals, and Cancer

You've known about cancer prevention agents, for example, nutrient C, lycopene, and beta-carotene, which are in numerous foods grown from the ground. Studies propose that individuals who eat dinners that are wealthy in leafy foods have a lower danger of malignant growth. An assortment of synthetic concoctions from plants known as phytochemicals likewise appear to shield cells from destructive mixes in food and in the earth, just as forestall cell harm and transformations, says Jed W. Fahey, ScD, MS, an associate teacher at Johns Hopkins Bloomberg School of Public Health and its School of Medicine who contemplates how cruciferous vegetables help secure against malady.

A diet that could avoid malignancy truly doesn't appear to be that unique from the solid foods you ought to eat at any rate, says Wendy Demark-Wahnefried, PhD, RD, associate chief for Cancer Prevention and Control at the University of Alabama's Comprehensive Cancer Center. That implies a lot of leafy foods, just as entire grains and lean meat or fish.

What's more, weight matters as well. Keep the scale at a solid number and shed a few pounds if required. Being overweight or hefty builds your danger of creating esophageal malignancy, postmenopausal bosom disease, colorectal disease, endometrial disease, ovarian disease, and others.

So, what foods would it be a good idea for you to stack up on to give your body the most obvious opportunity with regards to avoiding disease? WebMD examined investigate, at times clashing, to coax out certain foods you'll need to eat a lot of, beginning at this moment.

A bowl brimming with brilliant green steamed broccoli. You state either "Yum!" - Or "Where's the twofold cheeseburger?" But you realize the broccoli is beneficial for you, particularly without liquefied cheddar. The inquiry is, how acceptable? What's more, more to the point, can it - or any food - help forestall ailment, for example, malignancy?

The appropriate response is yes - a few foods do show malignant growth battling properties; however, nobody is yet ready to state some food can forestall or leave disease speechless. All things considered, an assortment of research recommends a general sound diet loaded up with brilliant products of the soil is the way to avoiding coronary illness, diabetes, and conceivably disease as well.

Truth be told, researchers find out about what not to eat - prepared meats, salty foods, sugary beverages, and gigantic helpings of red meat - than which leafy foods to heap on your plate. In any case, they do realize those foods matter.

A complete audit of thousands of concentrates on diet, physical movement, and weight directed for the World Cancer Research Fund and the American Institute for Cancer Research highlighted the advantages of eating for the most part foods of plant starting point. Foods, for example, broccoli, berries, and garlic indicated the absolute most grounded connections to disease avoidance.

They're low in calories and fat and force pressed with phytochemicals and cell reinforcements that may help lessen your malignant growth chance.

Cell reinforcements, Phytochemicals, and Cancer

You've known about cancer prevention agents, for example, nutrient C, lycopene, and beta-carotene, which are in numerous products of the soil. Studies recommend that individuals who eat dinners that are wealthy in leafy foods have a lower danger of malignancy. An assortment of synthetic substances from plants known as phytochemicals likewise appear to shield cells from hurtful mixes in food and in nature, just as forestall cell harm and transformations, says Jed W. Fahey, ScD, MS, an associate teacher at Johns Hopkins Bloomberg School of Public Health and its School of Medicine who examines how cruciferous vegetables help ensure against sickness.

A diet that could avoid disease truly doesn't appear to be that unique from the solid foods you ought to eat in any case, says Wendy Demark-Wahnefried, PhD, RD, associate chief for Cancer Prevention and Control at the University of Alabama's Comprehensive Cancer Center. That implies a lot of leafy foods, just as entire grains and lean meat or fish.

What's more, weight matters as well. Keep the scale at a solid number and shed a few pounds if required. Being overweight or corpulent expands your danger of creating esophageal disease, postmenopausal bosom malignancy, colorectal malignant growth, endometrial disease, ovarian disease, and others.

So, what foods would it be advisable for you to stack up on to give your body the most obvious opportunity with regards to avoiding malignant growth? WebMD investigated examine, at times clashing, to coax out certain foods you'll need to eat a lot of, beginning at this moment.

A bowl brimming with splendid green steamed broccoli. You state either "Yum!" - Or "Where's the twofold cheeseburger?" But you realize the broccoli is beneficial for you, particularly without liquefied cheddar. The inquiry is, how acceptable? Also, more to the point, can it - or any food - help forestall malady, for example, malignancy?

The appropriate response is yes - a few foods do show malignant growth battling properties; however, nobody is yet ready to state some food can forestall or leave disease speechless.

In any case, a group of research proposes a general solid diet loaded up with vivid leafy foods is the way to avoiding coronary illness, diabetes, and conceivably disease as well.

Actually, researchers find out about what not to eat - prepared meats, salty foods, sugary beverages, and colossal helpings of red meat - than which leafy foods to heap on your plate. Be that as it may, they do realize those foods matter.

A complete survey of thousands of concentrates on diet, physical action, and weight directed for the World Cancer Research Fund and the American Institute for Cancer Research highlighted the advantages of eating generally foods of plant source. Foods, for example, broccoli, berries, and garlic indicated probably the most grounded connections to disease anticipation.

They're low in calories and fat and force pressed with phytochemicals and cell reinforcements that may help lessen your disease chance.

Cell reinforcements, Phytochemicals, and Cancer

You've known about cancer prevention agents, for example, nutrient C, lycopene, and beta-carotene, which are in numerous foods grown from the ground. Studies recommend that individuals who eat dinners that are wealthy in products of the soil have a lower danger of malignant growth. An assortment of synthetics from plants known as phytochemicals likewise appear to shield cells from unsafe mixes in food and in the earth, just as forestall cell harm and transformations, says Jed W. Fahey, ScD, MS, an associate teacher at Johns Hopkins Bloomberg School of Public Health and its School of Medicine who contemplates how cruciferous vegetables help ensure against sickness.

A diet that could avoid malignant growth truly doesn't appear to be that unique from the sound foods you ought to eat at any rate, says Wendy Demark-Wahnefried, PhD, RD, associate chief for Cancer Prevention and Control at the University of Alabama's Comprehensive Cancer Center. That implies a lot of foods grown from the ground, just as entire grains and lean meat or fish.

Also, weight matters as well. Keep the scale at a sound number and shed a few pounds if required. Being overweight or large builds your danger of creating esophageal disease, postmenopausal bosom malignancy, colorectal malignancy, endometrial malignancy, ovarian malignant growth, and others.

So, what foods would it be a good idea for you to stack up on to give your body the most obvious opportunity with regards to avoiding disease? WebMD examined look into, at times clashing, to coax out certain foods you'll need to eat a lot of, beginning at the present time.

A bowl brimming with brilliant green steamed broccoli. You state either "Yum!" - Or "Where's the twofold cheeseburger?" But you realize the broccoli is beneficial for you, particularly without softened cheddar. The inquiry is, how acceptable? Furthermore, more to the point, can it - or any food - help forestall sickness, for example, malignancy?

The appropriate response is yes - a few foods do show malignant growth battling properties; however, nobody is yet ready to state some food can forestall or leave disease speechless. All things considered, an assemblage of research recommends a general sound diet loaded up with brilliant foods grown from the ground is the way to avoiding coronary illness, diabetes, and potentially disease as well.

Truth be told, researchers find out about what not to eat - handled meats, salty foods, sugary beverages, and colossal helpings of red meat - than which products of the soil to heap on your plate. Be that as it may, they do realize those foods matter.

A thorough survey of thousands of concentrates on diet, physical action, and weight led for the World Cancer Research Fund and the American Institute for Cancer Research highlighted the advantages of eating for the most part foods of plant beginning. Foods, for example, broccoli, berries, and garlic indicated the absolute most grounded connections to malignancy anticipation.

They're low in calories and fat and force pressed with phytochemicals and cell reinforcements that may help diminish your malignancy chance.

Cell reinforcements, Phytochemicals, and Cancer

You've known about cancer prevention agents, for example, nutrient C, lycopene, and beta-carotene, which are in numerous products of the soil. Studies recommend that individuals who eat suppers that are wealthy in leafy foods have a lower danger of disease. An assortment of synthetic concoctions from plants known as phytochemicals additionally appear to shield cells from hurtful mixes in food and in the earth, just as forestall cell harm and transformations, says Jed W. Fahey, ScD, MS, an associate teacher at Johns Hopkins Bloomberg School of Public Health and its School of Medicine who examines how cruciferous vegetables help secure against sickness.

A diet that could avert malignancy truly doesn't appear to be that unique from the sound foods you ought to eat in any case, says Wendy Demark-Wahnefried, PhD, RD, associate chief for Cancer Prevention and Control at the University of Alabama's Comprehensive Cancer Center. That implies a lot of leafy foods, just as entire grains and lean meat or fish.

Also, weight matters as well. Keep the scale at a solid number and shed a few pounds if required. Being overweight or stout expands your danger of creating esophageal disease, postmenopausal bosom malignant growth, colorectal malignant growth, endometrial disease, ovarian malignant growth, and others.

CONCLUSION

The Sirtfood diet was an achievement nourishment system a couple of years and was the dear eating routine with the broadsheet press at the time. In the event that you missed it, the features are that it incorporates red wine, chocolate, and espresso. Far less promoted and eye-catching, yet similarly uplifting news as we would like to think is the way that the response to the inquiry, 'would you be able to eat meat on the sirt nourishment diet? Is a resonating, yes?

The eating routine arrangement not just incorporates a decent sound part of the meat, it proceeds to recommend that protein is a basic consideration in a Sirtfood-based eating routine to receive the greatest reward.

We're not supporting this as some meat overwhelming eating routine we despite everything recollect the awful breath from Atkins, it's in reality very veggie-lover cordial and provides food for practically everybody, which is the thing that makes it so reasonable an alternative to us.

So, what is the Sirtfood diet? It was created by nutritionists Aidan Goggins and Glen Matten, following a pilot learn at the elite XK Gym, Daniel Craig, Madonna and an entire host of different celebs are supposedly individuals where they are the two experts in Sloane Square, London. Members in the preliminary lost 7lbs in the initial seven days, in what the creators call the hyper-achievement to organize. The science behind Sirtfoods drops out of an investigation in 2003 which found that a compound found in red wine, expanded the life expectancy of yeast. At last, this prompted the investigations which clarify the medical advantages of red wine, and how whenever drank reasonably individuals who drink red wine put on less weight.

A significant part of the science behind the Sirtfood diet is like that of 'fasting-diets' which have been well known for as far back as barely any years, whereby our bodies initiate qualities and our fat stockpiling is turned off; our bodies basically change to endurance mode, thus weight reduction. The negatives to fasting-eats fewer carbs are the unavoidable craving that results, alongside a decrease in vitality, bad-tempered conduct when you're "hungry", weariness and muscle misfortune. The Sirtfood diet professes to counter those negatives, as it's anything but a quick, so hunger isn't an issue, making it ideal for individuals who need to lead a functioning solid way of life.

Sirtfoods are a generally newfound gathering of nourishments that are incredible in actuating the 'sirtuin' qualities in our body, which are the qualities enacted in fasting eats fewer carbs. Critically for us carnivores, the guide proceeds to recommend in the section entitled 'Sirtfoods forever' that protein is basic to keep up digestion and decrease the loss of muscle when counting calories. Leucine is an amino corrosive found in protein, which praises and really upgrades the activities of Sirtfoods. This implies the most ideal approach to eat Sirtfoods is by consolidating them with a chicken bosom, steak or another wellspring of leucine, for example, fish or eggs.

Generally, we can thoroughly observe the advantage and intrigue of the Sirtfood diet. Like practically any eating regimen plan, it tends to be a faff getting every one of the fixings, and the 'Sirtfood green juice', which shapes a centerpiece of the initial 14 days of the arrangement, is a torment to make and really costly, yet it shows improvement over you'd anticipate. We just trialed a couple of days of the arrangement and keeping in mind that there was perceptible weight reduction, the genuine advantage is the reasonable methodology of bringing Sirtfoods into your regular dinner arranging.

Lightning Source UK Ltd.
Milton Keynes UK
UKHW050659150121
377099UK00003B/14